the evening of life

the evening of life

The Challenges of Aging and Dying Well

Edited by

JOSEPH E. DAVIS AND PAUL SCHERZ

University of Notre Dame Press
Notre Dame, Indiana

Copyright © 2020 by the University of Notre Dame
Notre Dame, Indiana 46556
undpress.nd.edu

All Rights Reserved

Published in the United States of America

Excerpts from W. B. Yeats's "Among School Children" and "Sailing to Byzantium" in chapter 4 are printed with the permission of Caitriona Yeats.

Library of Congress Control Number: 2020940875

ISBN: 978-0-268-10801-4 (Hardback)
ISBN: 978-0-268-10802-1 (Paperback)
ISBN: 978-0-268-10804-5 (WebPDF)
ISBN: 978-0-268-10803-8 (Epub)

CONTENTS

Acknowledgments vii

Introduction: Toward an Ethics of Aging   1
Joseph E. Davis

PART I. OUR DEFICIT MODEL OF AGING

ONE. The Devalued Status of Old Age   23
Joseph E. Davis

TWO. The Structural-Ethical Source of the Matter:
The Medical-Industrial Complex   38
Sharon R. Kaufman

THREE. Beyond Avoidance and Autonomy   46
Paul Scherz

PART II. LIVING OLD AGE WELL

FOUR. Epiphanies, Small and Large   67
Wilfred M. McClay

FIVE. The Contraction of Time and Existential Awakening:
A Phenomenology of Authentic Aging   78
Kevin Aho

SIX. The End of the Story: A Narrativist View of Life's Finale   94
Charles Guignon

SEVEN. Happiness and Aging: An Unlikely Combination?   105
Bryan S. Turner

PART III. AN OLD AGE THAT GOES WELL

EIGHT. Friendship, Citizenship, and Abandonment:
Older Adults with Dementia and without Family Caregivers   125
Janelle S. Taylor

NINE. The Priority of Social and Physical Function:
Older Adults in the CAPABLE Program   147
Sarah L. Szanton and Janiece Taylor

TEN. From Diagnosis to Person-Focused Prognosis:
Toward a Healthy Political Economy of Aging in America   161
Justin Mutter

Conclusion   181
Paul Scherz

Contributors   193

Index   197

ACKNOWLEDGMENTS

In March of 2018, we editors of this book held a conference on the ethics of later life at the Institute for Advanced Studies in Culture (IASC) at the University of Virginia. Many of the essays published as chapters here were first presented at that conference, with others prepared for this book. We owe a special debt to all of the conference participants. Given a storm that hit Virginia the day of the conference, many underwent heroic journeys just to be present. We thank those who prepared essays, including Thomas Pfau (whose paper is being published elsewhere), for their careful scholarship and generous responsiveness to the feedback of the conference discussants. The discussants were Anne Allison, Daniel Becker, Tal Brewer, James Mumford, China Scherz, and Jarrett Zigon. Their incisive comments on individual papers and vigorous engagement throughout the conference contributed much to the work that is found here.

We would also like to thank our colleagues in the Picturing the Human colloquy at the IASC—Tal Brewer, Matthew Crawford, and, especially, Justin Mutter—as well as Travis Pickell, for help in the initial work of conceptualizing the conference. The support of the IASC was critical, and, as always, we thank James Hunter and Ryan Olson. Kelly Blumberg provided first-rate administrative support and, along with Donita McCormick-Fortune and Vivienne Smith, saved the day with flexible and creative solutions to the many logistical challenges caused by the bad weather.

Kevin Aho, Wilfred McClay, and Bryan Turner were not able to attend the conference but subsequently prepared essays for this volume. This book is much stronger for their signal contributions.

We greatly appreciate the enthusiastic support of Stephen Wrinn, director of the University of Notre Dame Press, and for all his advice. We thank the three anonymous reviewers for the Press, from whose thoughtful and detailed comments we profited. And we would like to express our gratitude to Mariele Courtois for her careful editorial assistance and to Marilyn Martin of the Press for her graceful copyediting.

Immediately after the conference, somewhat more popular versions of the essays by Davis, McClay, and Mutter were published in the Fall 2018 number of the IASC's journal, *The Hedgehog Review*. We thank the editors of the *Review*, whose helpful editing was largely incorporated into the versions of the essays published here.

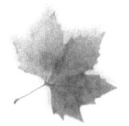

Introduction

Toward an Ethics of Aging

JOSEPH E. DAVIS

At other times and in other places, traditional ways of life, social classification, and metaphysical order gave shape and coherence to the course of life. The periods of aging, decline, and the approach of death were especially critical. They involve some of the most complex and unsettling aspects of human experience, and so the need for a defining community to provide direction and meaning was most acute. Many social and cultural practices, such as rites of passage, kinship networks, filial duties to ancestors, hierarchies that honor wisdom, social customs that superintend grief, and arts of suffering and dying, provided support and mediation for this time of life. In our "liquid times," by contrast, both in the Western world and beyond, common symbols and shared traditions of old age have weakened or disappeared altogether.[1] The meaning of the evening of life has become more subjective and private.

The task of preparing people for their later years, once a central cultural and philosophical task, has correspondingly waned. While the ideal form of character in the face of aging and death has varied by time and school of thought, social and cultural goals have nonetheless been broadly similar.[2] Social philosophies, religious communities, and civic cultures have helped guide people in a process of preparing for aging and dying "well." Such normative guidance and inspiration have not necessarily meant that old people have been given special respect or honor or that old age has been treated as a social category deserving of special treatment or public concern. Social histories tell an ambiguous story, with critical variation in respect accorded to different social groups.[3] But social norms of aging and dying did provide direction and shared expectations about how to live. One need only consider the many current debates that frame aging as a problem to be solved—with "successful aging," or anti-aging interventions, or "engineered negligible senescence,"[4] or assisted suicide—to see our communal and ethical quandary. We have precious few resources for even thinking about the enduring questions of a good old age, its meaning as a distinctive phase in the life course or stage in life's pilgrimage, and how we might prepare for and embrace the twilight years of life.

Our cultural impoverishment is rooted, most fundamentally, in a deficient conception of the person in society. Our dominant image of persons as free and unencumbered agents, as masters of choice, while inadequate at every stage of life, is especially detrimental in the last. Liberal, autonomous individualism provides virtually no criteria to inform our choices beyond personal preference. It situates us under a regime that effectively fixes aging and death as realities to hide; works to undermine our ability to cope with our finitude and inevitable decline; makes it difficult to sustain a valued sense of self in the face of dependency, disability, and an aging body; and works against a positive conception of living in older age. It is a regime that offers few grounds for social solidarity across the generations or reasons to strengthen it.

In our moment, the societies of the industrialized world urgently need an ethics of aging that centers on the question of a good human life in its later years—*an old age that is lived well and that goes well*.[5] Toward this ethics there are currently only scattered contributions.[6] Most of the existing literature might best be described as ethical reflections on issues that predominantly involve older people. This is an abstract ethics focused on rights, duties, and decision-making in legal matters and care in the context of formal institutions. It is not an ethics of everyday life for those navigating their twilight years. Of course, protections are crucial in hospitals, nursing homes, and other institutions where older people are especially vulnerable. An essential element of a good life is one in which people are treated justly, and an ethics of the person includes obligations.[7] But a substantive, normative ethics of aging must concern aging persons in all their complexity and must go beyond a concern with negative liberty. We need to re-envision a robust set of cultural concepts, practices, and virtues for advanced age and death, for individuals as well as communities. We need a positive image of living in old age, rooted in our shared *potentiality* and *vulnerability*, an image that engages our creativity and generativity juxtaposed with our frailty, our dependence, and our finitude. We need a holistic orientation to aging persons that is capable of guiding and delimiting interventions, whether medical or pertaining to quality of life. We need, in short, an ethics of aging that takes up conceptions of well-being in the evening of life and their complex interplay with the cultural frameworks, social arrangements, and technologies that impact those conceptions and might be shaped to sustain and satisfy them.[8]

Toward such an ethics, this book is an intervention.

Old Age as a Problem

No matter how we mark its beginning, "old age," as the English sociologist John Vincent has said, "is always the period of life before death."[9] The Danish philosopher Søren Kierkegaard called it the "evening of life," a time when life is beyond its afternoon but not yet at its nightfall.[10] Across history and across societies, what is meant by old age and at what point it commences varies considerably. Old age is a cultural category configured by kinship, economic systems, physical capacities, and basic value orientations rather than a stage defined in specific biological or chronological terms.[11] And it is not necessarily one period or status, but has often been divided into separate stages, as seen in the "ages of man" schemas of antiquity and medieval Europe, as well as various divisions of old age between an earlier, relatively healthy and independent "green" first phase and a frailer and more dependent later phase.[12] In our time, just such demarcations are sometimes labeled "young-old" and "old-old" or the "third age" and the "fourth age."[13] The end of old age, however, the last stage, is always that end that we call death. Its meaning is shaped by the growing shadow of death and the summation of all that has gone on before.[14]

Aging is both an individual and a social phenomenon. People are living longer than they used to, and because fewer children are being born, the population as a whole is aging. The age structure of most industrialized countries, which used to be in the shape of a pyramid, with relatively few people of old age at the top, is slowing becoming a rectangle, with the number of people alive at older ages slowly coming to mirror the number of those alive at younger ages.[15] According to the Census Bureau, the number of people age sixty-five and older in the United States now exceeds fifty million, accounting for more than 15 percent of the total population.[16] And that number will continue to grow steadily, as more than a third of the US population is now fifty or over.[17] In other countries, such as Japan, the population is aging even faster.[18]

Despite the fundamental importance of aging to life and the shifting demographics of society toward old age, there is a surprising dearth of ethical attention to aging. No field of moral inquiry is designated as an ethics of aging.[19] Such dilatory regard is even more remarkable when we consider the voluminous ethical literature on other domains of life, including reproduction, early life, and death. What might account for this gap? The short answer, I want to suggest, is the nearly complete absence of any positive, generative agenda. Not only do we lack a cultural framework for old age that is wider than the individual, as noted above,[20] but we also treat old age primarily as a social *problem*, approaching aged and dependent persons as ones to conceal or avoid. This stage of life is shrouded with an essentially negative veil, as many of the following chapters, beginning with Part I, will document.

In the face of an aging population, some speak of a "demographic time bomb" and "apocalyptic demography."[21] There is a pervasive worry that aging societies will be unproductive and create conflict over generational inequity. Urgent discussions are underway on a whole cluster of policy concerns centered on the allocation of resources. Healthcare access and distribution, the retiree safety net, and the "caregiver gap" are just some of the issues that have come to have greater social salience as the relative size of the population in old age has grown ever larger. According to the Alzheimer's Association, for example, "The number of Americans living with Alzheimer's is growing—and growing fast." As the population ages, so too will the number of new and existing cases.[22] In 1950, there were about seventeen workers supporting every beneficiary of Social Security; in 2013, there were fewer than three.[23] Because of divorce and smaller family sizes, the number of potential family caregivers to the older adults most in need (including family members, partners, or close friends) is shrinking dramatically.[24] These and other such developments in the United States and elsewhere have created a sense of crisis, casting aging and aging persons as dilemmas for others.

Our dominant cultural narratives of old age, especially but by no means only in the United States, are also negative, framed most commonly in terms of deficits. Our fluid, shifting culture and practice of liberal individualism make it particularly hard for us to face our finitude and identify with those who remind us of it. Much of what we mean by our celebrated "autonomy" is a form of social organization and policy that encourages us to live so as to repress and deny many features of the human condition, such as our dependence on the care of others and the vulnerability of our bodies. In so doing, we imagine that we are free of such realities, independent of those who sustain us, and even that we sit as the creators of the gifts we receive. This notion of autonomy provides no meaningful terms for expressing boundaries or limits or frailty or unchosen obligations or solidarity. It presupposes a kind of immortality in its explicit future orientation and in its implicit denial of the form given to life by the necessity of death.[25] This practice of detached self-sufficiency shapes how we envision ourselves and sets the norms and expectations by which we measure our experience and approach the world.

Reflecting this image and practice of autonomy, old age is typically viewed through either one of two contrasting cultural stories. On the one hand, we have a deprecating and frightening story of growing old, comprised of accounts of our steady deterioration, loss of control and dignity, and then ending, virtually imprisoned, with a medicalized death. There is reason to think that this common story, in light of both an aging population and medicalization, has intensified and increased age-stereotype negativity over time, not to mention the growing support for physician-assisted suicide.[26] The aged are "other" to us and even, as Kevin Aho notes in chapter 5, to our own future selves. On the other hand, we have an upbeat story of an ageless adulthood characterized by a continuation of activity, productivity, and good health throughout old age, followed by a brief decline and death. This second story, a liberation story told in both popular culture and in gerontological models such as "successful aging," is often contrasted with the first story, a loss narrative, and presented as a positive reappraisal of its negative and stereotypical terms. But it, too, as I'll argue in chapter 1, devalues old age as an unfortunate time of life, much inferior to youth. It, too, treats the period of growing old as a time without value in itself, offers no positive guidance for engaging dependence or vulnerability, and retains the same cultural antagonism to the aging body and approaching death.[27]

The growing medicalization of old age, proceeding within a logic that makes longevity an end in itself, does nothing to improve the picture. The aging person, when he or she appears to clinical medicine, does so only as a technical problem, in terms of a diagnosable illness or elevated risk factor. Medicine is dominated by an instrumental, problem-solving approach that affords professionals little time for attentive health *care* and frames even aging and the conditions of old age as challenges to be overcome with yet further interventions and increasing technical capacity.[28] In chapter 2, Sharon Kaufman shows just *how* the organization of ordinary medicine in the United States—its evidence base, standards of care, and reimbursement schemes—virtually forces doctors to recommend and older patients to receive ever more expensive and invasive treatments to address risk and extend life. Aimed at alleviating suffering, such treatments, used in a merely instrumental way without regard for what it means to be old, can cause great suffering. Turning our vaunted autonomy on its head, the self-perpetuating nature of technological medicine closes off alternatives because aging persons are not the subjects of concern, but their ailments or risks of adverse outcomes are.[29]

Both the successful aging model of gerontology and ordinary high-tech medicine embed ethical imperatives and an "implicit anthropology."[30] Though these fields present their ideas and practices as purely empirical matters—and thus as scientific and self-evident—they presuppose a background standard of what normal aging and the aging person are or should be. The presuppositions about being human in both fields share an evident alliance with those of liberal individualism—a picture of being human that deemphasizes or denies our temporality, our relationality, and the phenomenology of our vulnerable (and racialized, gendered, and classed) bodies. The standards valorize decision-making, full functioning, a voluntaristic model of relationships, and the self-interested fulfillment of preferences and plans. Any departure from the standard is a failure, such as a failure to "stay young" in the case of gerontology or to accept the "new obligation to longevity," as Kaufman calls it, in the case of medicine. Evaluation proceeds from concern with mental and bodily disorder rather than with retained or enhanced capacities.

When we move to our dominant ethical frameworks, we again encounter the basic anthropology of liberal autonomy and a deficit model of aging. As Paul Scherz shows in chapter 3, ethical approaches based on utilitarianism have little or nothing to say about aging persons qua aging persons, or, conversely and perhaps logically, they promote transhumanist dreams of the reversal or elimination of aging. Ethical approaches based on liberal proceduralism, such as bioethical principlism, are little better. Their concern is with formulating rules for professionals, who are enjoined, in the first instance, to respect the autonomous decision-making of patients and research subjects.[31] This limits the focus to a narrow range of specific policy matters, such as access to and quality of care, end-of-life decisions, advance directives, patient rights, and the like that are relevant to people of any age. They are not unique to older persons, and in these approaches there is a paucity of attention to old age as a distinctive and ethically salient phase of life. But in a deeper sense, the problem is with the notion of autonomy itself in "liquid times"—times without positive cultural resources for guiding our responses to aging and approaching death. Talk of "choice" for the aged can have only the thinnest formal meaning without commensurate attention to the larger social, medical, and normative context that actually confronts people as they age. And without an explicit anthropology of the constitutively relational, dependent, and embodied nature of persons, this approach, too, invites a view of aging as a deficit from a standard of self-sufficiency and control.[32] As Scherz argues, our foremost ethical theories lead to an avoidance of the lived realities of aging and preparation for death.

8 The Evening of Life

Living Old Age Well

For thinking about how to practice a good old age in community with others, our dominant cultural norms, our professional discourse ("successful aging") and practice (biomedicine), and our ethical theories fail us. We need something different, a form of ethics concerned with a good life and resourced from traditions, historical and cross-cultural, with richer anthropologies and meaningful frameworks for living old age. Scherz begins this reflection, sounding many of the themes that are carried further in Part II. He argues that the relational picture of humans at the heart of Christianity and many cultural systems provides positive accounts of the dependency and care, given and received, in aging and dying. These accounts offer hopeful alternatives to our shame at bodily weakness, fear of being a burden on others, and abhorrence of waning mental powers.[33] Further, Scherz argues, drawing on Buddhist, Christian, and Stoic sources, contemplation of death can help us develop the character dispositions we need to deal with the vicissitudes of old age and shape lives focused on higher goods.

The ethics of aging we need does not flinch from the realities of old age *and* draws out its distinctively valuable features. The crucial questions are both individual and social — What does it mean to live well in our later years? What features of our circumstances help our lives go well? In Part II we explore the first question, which is more than a matter of making old age a good part of life. It also includes reflection on the possibility, contra our culture and our ethicists, that there are goods to aging itself.[34] Like Scherz, the contributors to this part of the book, drawing on different traditions, affirm this possibility, rooted in a more adequate picture of the person and approaching death than our dominant cultural stories. All identify particular virtues and dispositions appropriate to growth in the evening of life, stress the value in suffering, and emphasize that an ethics of aging must necessarily be concerned with more than old age.[35] We are mortal by nature: We age throughout our life and can face its evening at any time. Living well at earlier ages will also have considerable impact on how we approach our later years and preparation for death. Moreover, these chapters affirm that speaking of goods of aging is not some unattainable ideal. Each contributor shows that we can learn from those older adults who already model adaptation and rich ways of being.

In chapter 4, Wilfred McClay asks, paraphrasing Yeats: How can the mounting debilities of old age be anything but a terrible sadness and pity? This is a decisive question for an ethics of aging, and we can only answer it, McClay argues, if we grasp and affirm what he aptly calls the paradox of human growth: "a startling play of reversals in which opposites trade places, and the loss of something ordinary becomes the path to the acquisition of something higher and rarer." Yes, old age can involve a veritable "carnival of losses," to quote the title of a book written by the poet Donald Hall as he neared ninety years of age.[36] But these losses can become gain, disability can become strength, if we open ourselves to certain truths of our temporality and the spirit. McClay calls these "epiphanies" because they come to us unbidden, and we often cannot know or understand the truth of them in advance, prior to some eliciting experience. When we are younger it is hard to imagine agedness as a finer thing, to see beyond mere appearance to the fuller completeness of all that a person is and has been. And in a cultural and commercial order, as I suggest in chapter 1, which always addresses us in terms of our preferences and plans, it is hard to imagine any quality to life, any sense of meaningful selfhood, that does not center on our self-mastery. Yet, as McClay shows, the adversities of old age, however great, can provide us with a deeper illumination of life, with a sense of wonder and a spirit enhanced, not diminished, by time and limitation. Even as we receive care, we can be a source of blessing to those around us.

In chapter 5, Kevin Aho, working from the tradition of existential phenomenology, draws out similar themes of temporality and cohesion, awakening and wonder. For the young and healthy, the horizon of the future is expansive, inviting initiative and exploration, and offering many potential paths for self-development. As we age, this horizon invariably begins to close in and grow foreshortened, closing off options and identities that are no longer livable. The simple truth is that we are vulnerable and circumscribed by time. We can deny this, or we can awaken to it. If received properly, Aho argues, the contraction of time and the losses and declines of aging, can present a new stage of life and new opportunities for personal and spiritual growth. This existential acceptance has the power to shake us out of the more superficial and trivial aspects of living, release us from ordinary fears of social rejection and failure, and free us for more sincere and honest forms of communication with loved ones.[37]

No longer taking our time for granted can help us accept stillness, grasp the preciousness of the moment, and unlock the wonder of seeing the world with fresh eyes. If received properly, the conditions of old age can give birth to a new, paradoxical, and authentic well-being, an experience we can see in the lives of many persons who have come to this acceptance.

In their respective ways, Scherz, McClay, and Aho all touch on the pivotal role of humility, gratitude, and acceptance in the face of aging, loss, and death and on the importance of our relationality, temporal unity, and capacity for wonder. In chapter 6, Charles Guignon elaborates on these qualities in light of a phenomenological (Heideggerian) picture of the social, situated human in the world. On this account, lives have a narrative structure, and Guignon seeks to develop an understanding of how we can be authentic to the overall shape of our story despite the challenges of old age and its particular mode of temporality. Especially in a youth-oriented culture, the evening of life is a time when we are depreciatively related to as old by others and often find the world around us growing less comprehensible and meaningful. Under these conditions, a well-lived old age, Guignon argues, requires the traits of resistance and forbearance. Resistance allows us to stay resolute, true to our narrative in the face of cultural influences and demeaning pressures. Forbearance allows us to accept the decline and dependence of old age—a "letting be" that can bring a resolution of our changing circumstances and adaptability to it while still holding onto our authentic life story. Together, resoluteness and acceptance can help us to live in old age with peace, reverence, and good humor.

In his review of contemporary ethics, Scherz notes that yet another school, that of virtue ethics, also has little to offer on aging and death because Aristotle, on whom it draws so heavily, provides no positive direction. In chapter 7, Bryan Turner confirms Aristotle's disparaging and logically inconsistent remarks about the possibility of flourishing in old age. But Aristotle's more general insights into the nature and context of human well-being, Turner suggests, can offer critical guidance for thinking about a good old age. First, Aristotle connects living well with habituation in virtue, which comes with time and through the life cycle, and, as an activity of the soul, can be lived and cultivated despite physical infirmities and decreasing capacities. Virtue prepares people for dealing with adversity and equips them with wisdom and a sphere of agency and control over themselves even in the face of temporal contraction and a dependency that Aristotle otherwise disparages. Second, Aristotle links flourishing inseparably to the practices of the wider community. This essential connection is often neglected in discussions of aging and happiness. As I note in chapter 1, reflection on loneliness among the aged typically ignores their social devaluation, isolation, or abandonment and emphasizes self-help. Similarly, as Turner shows, current reflection and theorizing about happiness is conducted in individualistic, passive, and hedonic/consumerist terms with little reference to the larger community or polity. But what Aristotle helps us to see, Turner argues, is that genuine well-being cannot be understood apart from social belonging.

An Old Age That Goes Well

An ethics of aging, as I noted above, must engage with the question of a good human life not only in terms of a life *lived well* in its later years but also in terms of a life that *goes well*. This second dimension, focused more explicitly on a vision of social solidarity and care, is the subject of Part III. Turner sets the stage by drawing out Aristotle's ethical thought on the contingency of life, our dependence on goods outside our control, and the social and political context necessary for human flourishing. From this perspective, well-being cannot be thought of or accessed in merely subjective (feelings of contentment) or material terms, much less simply as a matter of survival. Rather, for life to go well in old age we must attend to the actual challenges of embodiment and everyday life and to the condition of the wider social, political, and institutional environment upon which any meaningful sense of flourishing depends. The opportunity for a good old age, as the feminist literature on care has so clearly drawn out, is enabled or constrained by how we, as caregivers and as a community, treat our older citizens.[38]

The chapters in Part II focus on certain dispositions and virtues that are especially appropriate to adapting and living well in the evening of life. Each contributor notes some of the challenges discussed in Part I, particularly the cultural tropes and images that discount and diminish the aged. But while such devaluing representations are common and harmful, none is more unvarying or all-encompassing than the "catastrophizing" discourse about persons living with dementia or Alzheimer's disease.[39] Both professional and popular views are almost exclusively negative, framing dementia in heavily medicalized terms, as not only a loss of memory and ability but of selfhood and identity, a type of "living death."[40] Even when we are willing to talk of receptivity and adaptation in old age, of a value in and to aging and the last stage of life, we are tempted to draw the line at significant cognitive decline. Surely here we run up against the limit of speaking in any positive terms.

In fact, what we run up against are the limits of conceptualizing our personhood in narrowly individualistic and voluntaristic terms within an anthropology of ourselves as detached from others and in social relations put together by our choices and actions. What we need, as Janelle Taylor argues in chapter 8, is a better, more adequate picture, one that recognizes that we are beings-in-relationship, continuously sustained by supportive environments and practices of care. Since our selfhood is more than an individual property, the crucial question about living with dementia is not whether we lose selfhood but whether we lose the critical support of others who help sustain our selfhood. Empirical research is suggestive. One study, for example, found that while Alzheimer's disease does not bring about a loss of the person's "lifelong self," its maintenance requires the active support of care providers and family members.[41] So too, did another qualitative study find that persons living with dementia viewed the changes in the way they were treated by physicians, friends, and family as more damaging to their everyday well-being than the condition itself.[42]

What this means is that we cannot speak of life going well — a "best well" — without reference to a network of support and care, and this is acutely true and consequential for persons living with dementia. While family members normally form the first line of support, engaging kinship ties, for all the reasons discussed above, is growing more tenuous, and many of those in their later years find themselves alone. This situation is especially concerning for those with dementia, who form an increasing segment of the population without familial caregivers. If not from family, where can a supportive environment, one that sustains personhood, be found? One source, Taylor observes, is friends, either existing friends who stay connected and then take on greater roles of care after the onset of dementia or those who newly befriend a person with dementia who is without family support. Here again we see the role of small epiphanies and paradoxes in the face of sadness and loss. The challenge of friendship under these circumstances, Taylor shows, can open up new paths for *caregivers*, such as recognition of their own fundamental relationality, discovery of unsuspected dimensions in their friendship, personal growth and learning, and new skills of interpersonal interaction (see also chapter 9 on this point).

A relational understanding of persons and the need for the recognition of a supportive environment help us to see that care and caregiving are not voluntary matters and cannot be left to chance. They are community concerns, Taylor argues, and the community itself needs to be mobilized to better aid those giving and those receiving care. This support can, of course, take many forms, from changes to the legal system that impede nonfamily caregiving, as Taylor recommends, to the wider provision of natural and social primary goods. But with any such support, there is a critical need to avoid blanket assumptions about limitations and to engage and listen. Genuine care is a way of being attuned to persons, of responding to and affirming them in their wholeness and worth, of helping them establish an optimal relation to their own circumstances. This respect and concern cannot be programmed, reduced to rights, or carried on at a distance. It requires that we attend to the everyday experience of those in need, who must play as active a part as possible in defining what will be of help to them.

Care for persons living with dementia is a stark example of how an ethics of aging must engage with the inescapable realities and moral importance of embodiment. In most respects, of course, aging is a matter of the body. But far more than our biology, objectively conceived, is at stake. We *are* embodied. We experience our bodies, act in the world through our bodies, and are subject to many forces, social and material, that affect our bodies. All these aspects of our bodies are interrelated and have practical consequences for our health and well-being. Attending to embodiment, then, cannot be limited to a concern with symptoms and disease, but must extend to issues of living conditions, social disparities, access to care, personal relations, functional limitations, and more. As Sarah Szanton and

Janiece Taylor stress in chapter 9, for life to go well for older adults the whole embodied person must be brought into view.

The experience of aging, Szanton and Taylor argue, can be meaningfully enhanced by concentrating on challenging features of everyday life. Conversations with older people can easily show the activities that are actually valuable to them. Common priorities include aging in their own homes or neighborhoods, continued sociability through family and community involvement, the ability to look after themselves, and access to the simple pleasures of daily life. Enabling older persons to continue in these tasks for as long as possible is conducive to their quality of life, promotes resilience, and contributes to physical and emotional health, as well as being enriching to their families and communities. For the most part, what is needed to enhance this functionality, Szanton and Taylor show, is not sophisticated technology, but modest environmental modifications like stair rails, grab bars in showers and next to toilets, and better public transportation. They illustrate these insights with an unpretentious and highly effective program that enacts this person-centered, community-focused vision of care.

Just such a vision of care, attentive to the person and their everyday functioning, Justin Mutter argues in chapter 10, is a model for all of geriatrics. While a primary medical concern with physiology can be appropriate in the case of clearly identifiable diseases with known treatment regimes, it can become disastrous with age and growing *frailty*—with, that is, an increased complexity of health problems, functional limitations, and vulnerabilities. In the evening of life, good care must be directed to whole persons, with consideration of their lifeworlds, current circumstances, and resources, as well as specific health issues. As Mutter shows, there is considerable clinical and scientific evidence to demonstrate the effectiveness of whole-person care. Medicare, however, the insurance on which most older Americans depend, is based on a very different model, a model of testing and intervention that treats health as a sum of biological processes and directly links payment to those conditions, and only those conditions, that can be diagnostically coded. Rather than care directed to enhance overall functioning and reduce frailty, Mutter argues, Medicare requires the piecemeal and atomized treatment of individual illnesses.

In examining the political economy of Medicare, Mutter is arguing, like Kaufman in chapter 2, that a system based on an inadequate picture of older persons and their needs has become a source of harm. The single-minded and reductionistic focus on specific diagnoses has deep flaws, with little guarantee of actual improvement in health outcomes and a closing off of other potentially beneficial interventions. This type of harm is largely invisible to an ethics of abstract principles, procedure, and choice because the system of political economy structures, a priori, what options or courses of action are even available to physicians and patients. The choices, in effect, are already made. Instead of diagnosis, Mutter contends, funding should be tied to *prognosis*. This shift toward enhancing quality of life would allow for many of the insights developed in this book to be realized in medical care. It would focus on the whole person, on relational care, on global functioning, on limiting criteria—rather than warranting every incremental effort to extend life—and on developing a medical plan that takes the paradox of aging seriously.

Just at the time when many societies face unprecedented challenges to aging and dying well, we are unprepared. The common symbols, traditions, and ordering rituals that gave shape to people's life course and social meaning to their experience have nearly disappeared. Our ethical theories provide scant guidance for thinking about a good old age and preparing for death. Our growing technical capacities are not matched to an understanding of what it means to be old and so further blur the line between what is possible and what is good. Our dominant cultural stories, even the seemingly optimistic ones, frame a picture of the mounting debilities of old age as nothing but a terrible sadness and pity.

To find our way back to a robust set of cultural concepts and practices in advanced age, we need a positive picture of older adults that is capable of guiding us through decline and death. This requires a multidisciplinary effort, drawing on historical and cross-cultural sources, to better conceptualize and practice living and dying in the twilight of life, individually and collectively.

That is our goal in *The Evening of Life*. We propose a line of normative inquiry that begins with a picture of the human person in society that is richer than the liberal individualism of our cultural stories, dominant ethical systems, and medical practices. We turn to alternative philosophies and traditions to develop an interrelated set of conceptual tools, drawing on ideas of temporality, narrative, flourishing, and friendship, that can help us better understand the values and goods of aging and the last stage of life. We direct attention to the condition of the aged, to community practices and developments that exist to engage them and foster solidarity, and to the pressing need to explore how institutional systems work in practice. We work, in sum, toward illuminating our current predicament and charting a better way forward.

Notes

1. Zygmunt Bauman, *Liquid Times: Living in an Age of Uncertainty* (Cambridge: Polity Press, 2007).

2. See, for instance, Chris Gilleard, "Aging and Old Age in Medieval Society and the Transition of Modernity," *Journal of Aging and Identity* 7, no. 1 (March 2002): 25–41.

3. "Emerging out of the social and cultural history of old age at the beginning of the millennium is a strong awareness of the plurality of representations and experiences of old age over time and in any one time and place. It is more difficult to assess whether certain values concerning old age are more dominant at certain times and places than others, though we know enough to be wary of over-arching schema of cultural decline." Pat Thane, "Social Histories of Old Age and Aging," *Journal of Social History* 37, no. 1 (Autumn 2003): 93–111, 106.

4. Aubrey de Grey with Michael Rae, *Ending Aging* (New York: St. Martin's, 2007).

5. Much of the discussion here applies to the industrialized countries generally, though the programmatic responses in the third section of the book are addressed quite explicitly to a US context. We recognize that other areas of the world deal with aging differently, and that is a source of hope. See, for instance, Lawrence Cohen, *No Aging in India: Alzheimer's, the Bad Family, and Other Modern Things* (Berkeley: University of California Press, 1998). In framing an ethics of aging, we need to look both historically and cross-culturally for wider and richer perspectives.

6. Many of these contributions will be noted in the following chapters.

7. See, for instance, Rosemarie Tong, "Ethics of Aging," in *The International Encyclopedia of Ethics*, ed. Hugh LaFollette (Malden, MA: Blackwell, 2013), 1731–36.

8. This formulation draws on Michael S. McPherson, "Want Formation, Morality, and Some 'Interpretive' Aspects of Economic Inquiry," in *Social Science as Moral Inquiry*, ed. Norma Haan, Robert N. Bellah, Paul Rabinow, and William M. Sullivan (New York: Columbia University Press, 1983), 96–124, 112.

9. John Vincent, *Old Age* (London: Routledge, 2003), 132.

10. Søren Kierkegaard, *Three Discourses on Imagined Occasions*, ed. and trans. Howard V. Hong and Edna H. Hong (Princeton, NJ: Princeton University Press, 1993), 56.

11. Of course, in many bureaucratic contexts, such as retirement from paid labor or access to pension plans, chronological age is used.

12. Thane, "Social Histories of Old Age and Aging," 99.

13. Jacquelyn Boone James and Paul Wink, "The Third Age: A Rationale for Research," in *Annual Review of Gerontology and Geriatrics*, vol. 26: *The Crown of Life: Dynamics of the Early Postretirement Period*, ed. Jacquelyn Boone James and Paul Wink (New York: Springer, 2006), xix–xxxii.

14. "Old age is the period of life when the shape of life as a whole comes into view, or when it is natural, at any rate, to try to see things in a wider scale." Harry R. Moody, "The Meaning of Life in Old Age," in *Aging and Ethics*, ed. Nancy S. Jecker (New York: Humana Press, 1991), 51–92, 57.

15. See, for example, S. Jay Olshansky, "The Demographic Transformation of America," *Daedalus* 144, no. 2 (Spring 2015): 13–19.

16. US Census Bureau, "The Nation's Older Population Is Still Growing, Census Bureau Reports," June 22, 2017, https://www.census.gov/newsroom/press-releases/2017/cb17-100.html.

17. US Census Bureau, https://censusreporter.org/profiles/01000US-united-states/.

18. For World Bank data on the percentage of the population over 65 for every country, see World Bank, https://data.worldbank.org/indicator/SP.POP.65UP.TO.ZS?view=chart.

19. Christopher Simon Wareham, "What Is the Ethics of Ageing?" *Journal of Medical Ethics* 44, no. 2 (February 2018): 128–32, 128. In his Introduction to *The Palgrave Handbook of the Philosophy of Aging*, editor Geoffrey Scarre writes: "'Old age is a topic that philosophers by and large have ignored,' said [Mary] Mothersill in 1999; and a decade and a half later the situation remains largely unchanged" (London: Palgrave Macmillan, 2016), 1–10, 2.

20. Moody, "The Meaning of Life in Old Age," 52.

21. Ann Robertson, "The Politics of Alzheimer's Disease: A Case Study in Apocalyptic Demography," *International Journal of Health Services* 20, no. 3 (July 1990): 429–42.

22. Alzheimer's Association, "2018 Alzheimer's Disease Facts and Figures," https://www.alz.org/alzheimers-dementia/facts-figures.

23. See the Social Security history at Social Security Administration, "Social Security History," https://www.ssa.gov/history/ratios.html.

24. Donald Redfoot, Lynn Feinberg, and Ari Houser, "The Aging of the Baby Boom and the Growing Care Gap: A Look at Future Declines in the Availability of Family Caregivers," *Insight on the Issues*, AARP Public Policy Institute 85 (August 2013).

25. As the sociologist Georg Simmel once wrote, "In every single moment of life we *are* those who must die, and each moment would be different if this were not in effect our predetermined condition" (emphasis in original). In "The Metaphysics of Death," *Theory, Culture & Society* 24, nos. 7–8 (December 2007 [April 1910]): 72–77, 74.

26. Reuben Ng, Heather G. Allore, Mark Trentalange, Joan K. Monin, and Becca R. Levy, "Increasing Negativity of Age Stereotypes across 200 Years: Evidence from a Database of 400 Million Words," *PLoS One* 10, no. 2 (February 2015): e0117086. The authors write, "We found that age stereotypes have become more negative in a linear way over 200 years. In 1880, age stereotypes switched from being positive to being negative. In addition, support was found for two potential explanations. Medicalization of aging and the growing proportion of the population over the age of 65 were both significantly associated with the increase in negative age stereotypes."

27. I also discuss the anti-aging movement, which treats aging in purely biological terms and as something that can be postponed or eliminated.

28. On the "fix" orientation of medicine, see Joseph E. Davis and Ana Marta González, eds., *To Fix or to Heal: Patient Care, Public Health, and the Limits of Biomedicine* (New York: New York University Press, 2016).

29. The physician Atul Gawande, reflecting on his dying father's desire to go home, notes this conundrum: "In a hospital built to ensure survival at all costs and unclear how to do otherwise, he [his father] understood his choices would never be his own." *Being Mortal* (New York: Metropolitan, 2014), 253.

30. Søren Holm, "The Implicit Anthropology of Bioethics and the Problem of the Aging Person," in *Ethics, Health Policy and (Anti-) Aging: Mixed Blessings*, ed. Maartje Schermer and Wim Pinxten (Dordrecht: Springer Netherlands, 2013), 59–71.

31. See "Chapter 4: Respect for Autonomy" from the leading textbook of principlism, Tom L. Beauchamp and James F. Childress, *Principles of Biomedical Ethics*, 7th ed. (New York: Oxford University Press, 2013), 101–40. According to critical gerontologists Martha Holstein and Mark Waymack, "With a few im-

portant exceptions, to applied ethicists choice . . . is what matters" (references deleted). From "The Contributions of Philosophy and Ethics in the Study of Old Age," in *Enduring Questions in Gerontology*, ed. Debra J. Sheets, Dana Burr Bradley, and Jon Hendricks (New York: Springer, 2006), 177–201, 182.

32. See also the discussion in Holm, "The Implicit Anthropology of Bioethics."

33. These are all concerns nowhere more sharply expressed than in the growing call for assisted suicide. As an example, see Norman L. Cantor, "On Avoiding Deep Dementia," *Hastings Center Report* 48, no. 4 (August 2018): 15–24.

34. See the discussion in Frits de Lange, "Imagining Good Aging," in *Ethics, Health Policy and (Anti-) Aging: Mixed Blessings*, ed. Maartje Schermer and Wim Pinxten (Dordrecht: Springer Netherlands, 2013), 135–46.

35. Georg Simmel, writing in 1910, notes, "Just as we are hardly already present at the moment of our birth, but rather something is continuously being born from us, so too do we hardly die only in our last moment. . . . Death limits, that is, it gives form to life, not just in the hour of death, but also in continually colouring all of life's contents." In "The Metaphysics of Death," 74.

36. Donald Hall, *A Carnival of Losses: Notes Nearing Ninety* (New York: Houghton Mifflin Harcourt, 2018).

37. See further Paul Scherz, "Living Indefinitely and Living Fully: Laudato Si' and the Value of the Present in Christian, Stoic, and Transhumanist Temporalities," *Theological Studies* 79, no. 2 (May 2018): 356–75.

38. See, among many sources, Marian Barnes, *Care in Everyday Life: An Ethic of Care in Practice* (Bristol: Policy Press, 2012), and Liz Lloyd, "Mortality and Morality: Ageing and the Ethics of Care," *Ageing and Society* 24, no. 2 (March 2004): 235–56.

39. Peter Reed, Jennifer Carson, and Zebbedia Gibb, "Transcending the Tragedy Discourse of Dementia: An Ethical Imperative for Promoting Selfhood, Meaningful Relationships, and Well-Being," *AMA Journal of Ethics* 19, no. 7 (July 2017): 693–703.

40. Elizabeth Peel, "'The Living Death of Alzheimer's' versus 'Take a Walk to Keep Dementia at Bay': Representations of Dementia in Print Media and Carer Discourse," *Sociology of Health & Illness* 36, no. 6 (July 2014): 885–901.

41. Sam Fazio, *The Enduring Self in People with Alzheimer's: Getting to the Heart of Individualized Care* (Baltimore, MD: Health Professions Press, 2008).

42. Reed et al., "Transcending the Tragedy Discourse of Dementia."

PART I

Our Deficit Model of Aging

CHAPTER ONE

The Devalued Status of Old Age

JOSEPH E. DAVIS

In our society, old age is understood and addressed in ways that lead inevitably to its devaluation. Its status is low and arguably is falling. On its face, such a claim might sound preposterous. Surely, the opposite is true. From the Social Security safety net to the Americans with Disabilities Act, from the positive portrayals of older people in popular media to near-record life expectancy, this is unquestionably the golden age of the golden years, a time of "No Limits. No Labels," to quote a slogan of the American Association of Retired Persons (AARP). The scope of identification with the aged is wide, this time of life is treated with public respect, and extensive supports and accommodations for living well are provided. By what blinkered perspective or romanticization of the past can we fail to see this obvious progress?

There have been a great many improvements to the material welfare and health of the aged, no question of that. But there is another feature of our present situation, loudly touted as a breakthrough, that I want to argue is actually counterproductive and contributes to a devaluation rather than an enhancement of the evening of life. What I have in mind are the "new positive images of aging," which, according to the sociologist Stephen Katz, "depict activity, autonomy, mobility, choice, and well-being in defiance of traditional gloomy stereotypes of decline, decrepitude, and dependency."[1] These new images create their own expectations and obligations and deny the last stage of life its own meaning and character. And without those, old age can have no valued standing.

The evening of life is being redefined by imperatives that are not in themselves new, but are increasingly pressed onto the aged. One such force is the concern with the viability of public programs that provide income and health insurance for the elderly. Underlying much of this concern, and the resulting public discussion, are a growing sense of fiscal crisis and calls for cost-cutting reforms. The subsequent formulation of economic priorities and policies on aging is, in turn, amplifying another force that is engulfing old age: the growing medicalization of the lives of older adults. Efforts to fight rising costs are both informing and working in tandem with new and inflexible duties of health surveillance, prevention efforts, and lifestyle changes.

The trend toward medicalization dovetails with yet a third force, the commercialization of old age. Commercialization is inciting and informing imperatives to optimize self and body, realized through vast new industries of goods and services, including anti-aging interventions. Public policy, medicalization, and commercialization: All of these forces and more are generating new standards for and expectations of old age and contributing to its devaluation.

But a devalued old age cannot be explained solely by economic, medical, or commercial pressures. The challenge goes deeper. It involves basic cultural orientations—to time, kinship, social organization, the transcendent, and value premises about what it is good to do and good to be. We find ourselves today with a construction of old age built according to an irredeemable cultural logic.[2] That logic and its inevitable consequences become clear in various representations of old age and aging that I briefly consider. One is representations of aging in popular culture. In this sphere, vitality, fitness, and productivity, no matter the age, are the measures of aging well. The second case involves representations of aging in the gerontological discourse of "successful aging" and in anti-aging medicine. In these discourses, normal aging and death are implicitly or explicitly defined as a failure. And, finally, I want to consider representations of aging in the rhetoric of concern about a growing "epidemic of loneliness." In an important sense, the aged disappear in this discourse as their lifeworlds and vulnerabilities are reduced to individualized, medicalized problems.

Outside Time and Finitude

The last decade has seen the emergence of a plethora of health, fashion, and lifestyle blogs aimed at people over fifty or sixty years of age: *Atypical Sixty, Fabulous over Sixty, Age Is Just a Number, Muddling through My Middle Age, Second Lives Club*, and so on. Typically run by one or two individuals, the blogs and vlogs create an audience and interactive community around the discussion of aspects of living in one's older years. Many also generate revenue by deftly acting as intermediaries between their audiences and commercial enterprises that support the sites.[3]

For a window on popular norms of aging, I chose *Sixty and Me*, a "community of 500,000 women over 60," founded by Margaret Manning. Not only does the site claim to have a very large following, but it also covers a wider range of topics than most, including health, travel, money, life, mindset, dating, and beauty. *Sixty and Me* further recommends itself with its mainstream tone and advice. There are sites offering fanatical fitness regimes, calorie restriction diets, and "senior sex news," but this is not one of them.

Sixty and Me brims with advertising. Manning is the central figure, but there are also many contributions by various experts, typically with something to sell. While there is some discussion of caregiving, self-care for caregivers, and the need to talk about death, there is little mention of suffering, decline, or death itself. These topics, it seems, don't translate well into advertising opportunities. As gerontologist Harry Moody once observed about marketing to the older demographic: "The appeal is always to turn away from outdated images of maturity in favor of reinvented identity outside of time and finitude."[4]

At *Sixty and Me*, an appeal to emancipation and reinvention informs the picture of good aging. That picture draws on familiar American norms of an independent, self-sufficient, and enterprising self. In one showcased post, for example, Manning quotes the actor Jamie Lee Curtis, then fifty-six: "If I can challenge old ideas about aging, I will feel more and more invigorated. I want to represent this new way. I want to be a new version of the 70-year-old woman. Vital, strong, very physical, very agile. I think that the older I get, the more yoga I'm going to do."[5]

In commenting on Curtis and on this quote, Manning makes three points. She notes that Curtis "isn't afraid of getting older. Instead of seeing life after 60 as a time to take it easy, she is looking forward to the opportunity to make the absolute most of her life." Manning adds that she appreciates "the fact that Jamie Lee Curtis realizes that, as a celebrity, she has a role to play in challenging aging stereotypes." And finally, Manning approvingly observes that Curtis "calls attention to the fact that life after 50 is a choice. At 56, Curtis is already planning for the decades ahead. As she correctly points out, the older she gets, the harder she will need to work to maintain her energy and physical strength."

Make the most of life, live so as to challenge "old ideas about aging," and treat life after fifty (or sixty or seventy) as a choice: These are the three norms that Manning takes Curtis to be living by and that Manning finds "right on the money," as do many (though certainly not all) of the blog readers who commented on the article since its initial posting. In this view, later life should not be a time for less engagement or a reorientation away from a view of the world as a task zone, but rather a period of continual goal-seeking, work, or other contributive role-taking. The future is open, inviting, ready to reward new initiatives.

This liberal individualist picture of people as independent agents, masters of their lives through volition and choice, is familiar. As social institutions have declined in recent decades, however, there has been an even greater emphasis on self-optimization. The language for expressing this imperative has taken a number of forms since the 1960s, with terms like human potential, positive thinking, empowerment, "peak performance," and self-esteem variously in use. A prominent rubric that began to spread in the 1980s framed autonomous persons as "enterprising" people energetically striving, with calculation and efficiency, to project a future and act to achieve their goals.[6] The notion that life after fifty is a choice and is anything we want to make of it brings together the norm of self-optimization—Curtis will not be retiring or taking it easy, but making the absolute most of her life—with two related and widely accepted ideas: that health is an achievement and that body image is an integral component of personal identity.[7] All of these ideas meet in the joint concept of "health and fitness," which is presented by Curtis as the decisive blow to the old stereotypes of aging. What will make Curtis a "new version of the 70-year-old woman" is the fit and vital body that she will work ever harder to produce.

Aging well by such criteria, as the outcome of choices, requires continuous demonstrations of success through signs of initiative and energy. Appearance—looking healthy, fit, and "put together"—is also crucial: "To look old is to be old."[8] In the comments section of *Sixty and Me*, people sometimes report on how they look younger than they are. As one reader put it, "I am 70 (even though most folks tell me I look at least 10 years younger)." Such self-affirmation signals that they are aging well.

Another example illustrates this performative quality. In a discussion of "fashion for women over 60," Manning stresses looking "fabulous without trying to look younger." One of her fashion secrets is to "embrace your age." Elaborating on that advice, she writes that "when people try to dress in styles that would be more appropriate for someone much younger, they paradoxically make themselves look much older. . . . If you "dress age appropriately," it often has the effect of making you look younger because people are not distracted by age-inappropriate clothing, and instead can appreciate what great shape you're in, or how healthy your skin is, or what a stylish haircut you have."[9]

Again, the measure is the body. Health, fitness, a youthful appearance, entrepreneurial energy: These are not "add-ons," like fashion or cosmetics; they are something you *are*. The point of the advice of *Sixty and Me* is not so much to deny the aging process as to postpone it to some indefinite future. The message is that good aging is living later life as if you were young, though with a necessarily even more exacting regimen of diet, exercise, and risk reduction practices—and, given that this good aging is a matter of choice and responsibility, with the unspoken implication that problems and failures are self-inflicted.

Personal efforts to stay fit or engage in work are certainly not to be derided. What is of concern is the language of individual choice, the incitement to a self-optimization understood in terms of "productivity" and an open future, and the use of the body as an instrument to register a superior position. There are no grounds here for coping with disability and decline, physical or mental, or for embracing old age as a valued and dignified final chapter in its own right. And in the individualism being promoted there is precious little rationale for interdependence: for the humility, for instance, to accept care or the commitment to provide it. Despite the effort to project a positive image, what is on offer is a construction of old age that can only intensify and perpetuate its devalued status.

The "New Gerontology"

The picture of aging that comes through on *Sixty and Me* has been a feature of consumer culture for decades. But in the late 1980s, it entered mainstream gerontology. The leading theorists of the "new gerontology," John Rowe and Robert Kahn, distinguished their vision of positive aging from the "negative perspective" of the old gerontology and the "myths" and "denial" of society at large.[10] Previously, gerontologists had treated age-related alterations in physical and cognitive functioning that were not due to disease or disability as normal and inevitable and unassociated with lifestyle and risk. Rowe and Kahn, by contrast, argued that many characteristics of and age-related disease risks were related to lifestyle and other environmental factors and that much of the decline in older age was therefore avoidable. With the right choices and the discipline to follow a careful regime of risk reduction, individuals could attain "successful aging," generally characterized in the gerontological literature as sustained health and vitality in the later years.

Success, in those terms, means living with little disease or disability, maintaining high levels of cognitive and physical functioning, and remaining active and independent for as long as possible.[11] In an important sense, you satisfy the criterion of "successful" only to the degree that you are not "old."[12] If you are frail, functionally disabled, disengaged, or have health risks, such as high blood pressure, your aging is "usual." That doesn't sound so bad, but, as many critics have pointed out, the opposite of success is not "usual." It is "failure."[13]

The normative appeal of the new gerontology to individual autonomy and responsibility makes it even clearer that "failure" is precisely what is at stake.[14] Health is a matter of individual choice, and it becomes each person's moral duty to muster all of his or her energies to be successful. Insufficient initiative, insufficient efforts to stay informed, incomplete compliance with expert advice, and the like are grounds for potential blame, stigmatized as fatalism and passivity and made the target of interventions by others. Calling, and getting called, to account for any slacking has become a pervasive phenomenon, so common that we offer anticipatory apologies when we know that others know that we have done anything less than prioritize our health and longevity. There are no excuses.

The popularity of the successful aging model and its imperatives has, predictably, contributed to the steep rise in the use of anti-aging therapies.[15] If old age is open and indefinite and aging is a choice and a technical challenge, pursuing such interventions for the sake of "success" would seem not only fitting but obligatory.

Anti-aging is big business.[16] By far the most common and commercially profitable components are those interventions that help hide, postpone, or compensate for the effects of aging on the body.[17] Anti-wrinkle cream and Botox disguise and conceal; fitness programs and nutritional supplements stave off decline; Viagra and hormone replacement therapy compensate or reinvigorate. Most such interventions are readily available, including the more compensatory, through the growing phenomena of specialty longevity clinics, sometimes known as anti-aging centers or life extension institutes.[18]

Restorative medicine is one aspect of a larger anti-aging medicine and science. Interventions that might slow the aging process and extend the human lifespan are being pursued through research into genetics, the biochemistry of cellular senescence, and stems cells. Optimism about this enterprise has been bolstered by successful efforts to manipulate the longevity of nematode worms, fruit flies, and mice.[19] Some now believe that the human lifespan can be extended twenty to sixty years. Even further out on the edges of longevity research are some provocateurs who claim that aging can be stopped and even reversed. These are members of what the philosopher Mary Midgley aptly calls the "new immortalist movement"[20] — new in its invocation of science, though this movement can claim a long and storied lineage.[21]

Anti-aging research goes further than gerontology in medicalizing aging itself, defining it as a condition of degeneration, a technical failure that can be technically modified. And it promotes interventions, such as hormone treatments, that gerontology rejects as unproven and dangerous, and it does so for people who may be without clinical impairment or even elevated risk. Despite their differences, however, anti-aging and successful aging push toward a similar framing of old age as undesirable and, at least for a time, preventable. Both treat frailty and disability as indications of failure and emphasize individual choice and effort without regard to the hardships and inequalities that many older people actually endure.[22] Both promote an evasion of the inevitable confrontations with disability, disease, and death. Both stoke insatiable and unwarranted expectations of medicine and undermine the grounds for accepting limits and reconciling ourselves to what cannot be changed. To paraphrase Ivan Illich on coping with pain, only aging perceived as controllable or curable is felt to be intolerable.[23]

Under the paradigm embraced by proponents of both successful aging and anti-aging, old age has no value in itself. "Old" signifies bodily decline, while "success" involves a ceaseless battle to defeat degeneration, and hope is always invested in the prospect of overcoming limits through self-reliance and technological interventions. There is no space here for stillness or release, no sense of value or consolation in the evening of life. Even cultivating spirituality is framed instrumentally in terms of promoting "better physical and mental health in old age."[24] An imperative to defeat aging and even death can only consign these realities to fear, shame, and avoidance.

Further, and for the same reason, situating aging in a framework of success and failure, or victory and defeat, helps undermine the social basis for care and solidarity. Fear and avoidance contribute to the isolation and marginalization of the old, infirm, and dying. It is already difficult for those with little experience of aging or infirmity to empathize with it, and those younger and of good health are often and understandably motivated to avoid the idea of their own decline and death. Representations of old age that add censure and shame to greater dependence and loss of one's powers can only make matters worse.

An Epidemic of Loneliness

There is no sugarcoating the experience of aging, in our day or any other. For instance, in a sermon on the "infirmities and comforts of old age," first published in 1805, the seventy-five-year-old pastor of a Congregationalist church in Massachusetts lays out key virtues and a role of spiritual service for the aged. But first he provides a sober description of old age as "a time when strength faileth." As we age, he observes, we experience a decay of our bodily strength: "Our customary labor becomes wearisome . . . pains invade our frame . . . our sleep, often interrupted, refreshes us less than heretofore . . . our food is less gustful . . . our sight is bedimmed, and our ears dull of hearing." Along with all this and mental decline, the pastor notes, we often experience a gradual loss of companions and social visits and an increase in isolation. Moreover, to our disadvantage, "we contrast our present with our former condition" of active powers, and "not only the remembrance of what is past, but the forethought of what is to come, aggravates the calamity of the aged man."[25]

In *The Loneliness of the Dying*, the sociologist Norbert Elias argues that, over time, these weakened bonds and other common features of the later years have been compounded by increased individualization and the isolation of the "ageing and dying from the community of the living." In contemporary society, Elias argues, older persons are "pushed more and more behind the scenes of social life," a process that intensifies their devaluation, emotional seclusion, and loss of social significance. A physical and institutional sequestering and a pervasive cultural tendency to "conceal the irrevocable finitude of human existence" have made it harder for them and those around them to relate to, understand, and interact with one another. The aged and dying are less likely to receive the help and affection they need, and they are more prone to different forms of loneliness and painful feelings of irrelevance. "Never before," Elias writes, "have people died as noiselessly and hygienically as today in [more developed] societies, and never in social conditions so much fostering solitude."[26]

In recent years, the loneliness of the aged has received increasing public attention, sometimes under the rubric of an "epidemic of loneliness." While this "epidemic" affects people at every age, much of the discussion of it, especially proposed responses, tends to focus on the elderly. Popular articles and books identify a number of social changes as contributing factors.

Among these are high divorce rates, including a steady uptick in after-fifty "gray divorce," smaller families and extended-family networks, more single-member households, and fewer opportunities for social activities.

Contributors to the public discussion frame loneliness itself as a kind of medical condition or disorder: It is something one "suffers from," that is partly heritable, that has characteristic "symptoms" and "risk factors," can become "chronic," and needs to be "treated." Like other animals, such as fish, mice, and prairie voles, we "evolved to be social creatures," these writers remind us. Therefore, literally fatal consequences can result from our "perception of isolation from others—of being on the social perimeter," to quote social neuroscience popularizers John and Stephanie Cacioppo. Our "perceived social isolation," the two neuroscientists write, "can still put us in self-preservation mode," a "hangover" from our evolutionary past that is now "at odds with thriving in a modern society." Like a lack of social ties, identified by Rowe and Kahn as a threat to health, loneliness is found to have detrimental effects on "long-term health and well-being." For example, Vivek Murthy, a former US surgeon general, reports that loneliness and isolation are "associated with a reduction in lifespan similar to that caused by smoking 15 cigarettes a day and even greater than that associated with obesity."[27]

In discussions of loneliness and how to "solve" this problem, virtually the entire focus is on its harmful consequences for health and longevity. These appear to be the values that really matter, and the evidently urgent need to address the epidemic flows from concerns with this harm and the costs it imposes on society. Health and longevity are the ends to which remedial action is directed and by which outcomes are evaluated. Even in discussions that include exhortations to build strong connections and communities, loneliness and isolation are treated as individual conditions, and references to community easily coexist with talk of genetic hardwiring, the role of the prefrontal cortex, and the ways in which neural mechanisms might generate feelings of loneliness. Readers are reassured that researchers are hard at work "deepening their understanding of [loneliness's] biological underpinnings."[28] The hope, it seems, is that we can get rid of that "hangover" and stop feeling so much distress in the face of loneliness and social isolation. A psychoactive drug for loneliness might be a start, on which possibility, John and Stephanie Cacioppo note, "animal research is shedding light."[29]

Health consequences are a legitimate concern, of course, but this medicalized discourse of loneliness barely touches on the actual social conditions and vulnerabilities of the aged. Little or nothing is said of their practical challenges in everyday life, their loss of social significance, their isolation from the community, or their abandonment. In fact, the definitions of the "epidemic" often downplay, if not effectively deny, that the social fabric and our mutual dependence are even at issue. Many of the recommended strategies to reduce loneliness place the burden on the lonely themselves. Typical advice is often some form of self-help: take a class, get a dog, volunteer, build your confidence with social skills training, seek out behavioral therapy. With therapy—highlighted for its positive "impact"—the aged lonely can be helped to see that their low self-worth, perceived isolation, or feelings of being unwanted are probably just cognitive errors that need to be "restructured." Once this restructuring is accomplished, the aged can better match what they want in social life with what they have and get on with aging more successfully. The status quo can now appear in a new, more uplifting light. The larger world and the incomparable meaning of the company of others for people need scarcely be acknowledged.[30] The aged, ostensibly the subject of concern, disappear.[31]

More than a "Pitiful Appendage"

The psychologist Carl Jung once observed that "a human being would certainly not grow to be seventy or eighty years old if this longevity had no meaning for the species. The afternoon of human life must also have a significance of its own and cannot be merely a pitiful appendage to life's morning."[32]

If old age is to be more than a "pitiful appendage," we need a way of relating to ourselves, our life-course, and death that gives genuine significance to getting older. Current constructions of old age in individualistic terms of self-reliance, the fit body, productive accomplishments, or an imperative to deny or defeat aging technologically cannot but deepen our predicament and the need to render it invisible. This is what makes the cultural logic of these constructions irredeemable. They leave us in a cul-de-sac, hemmed in by a predatory commercial culture, a punishing ideology of health, fewer and weaker social ties, an ethic of active striving and mastery, and a mechanistic picture of ourselves. Moving beyond the devaluation of old age requires other orientations and other practices for which we must look elsewhere—to other societies, past or present, and to older traditions.

We know, from history, theology, philosophy, and anthropology, that there *are* other possibilities. The temporal orientation need not be toward an open, this-worldly future, but toward wisdom, narrative, memory, and, for people of faith, a future that is eternity. The social orientation of the evening of life need not be individualistic, but toward family and the localization and strengthening of social relations. Similarly, the view of the life cycle need take its bearings not from youth and middle age, but from roles and identities appropriate to old age, with their own norms and rewards. These norms and rewards need not be defined in terms of active striving and productivity, but in terms of release, such as from social climbing, and a more contemplative attitude toward the world. Surely, in the last stage of life, health and longevity need not continue to be treated as ends in themselves. Rather, they might be set within a larger framework of limits, a recognition of our vulnerability and dependence, and the ethic of a well-lived life. There *are* other possibilities, and if we are to free ourselves from the iron cage to which our cultural logic consigns us, we need to look to them for direction.

Notes

1. Stephen Katz, "Growing Older without Aging? Positive Aging, Anti-Ageism, and Anti-Aging," *Generations* 25, no. 4 (Winter 2001–2002): 27–32, 27.

2. I borrow this phrase from John Vincent, who uses it in the narrower context of anti-aging medicine. See Vincent, "What Is at Stake in the 'War on Anti-Ageing Medicine'?," *Ageing and Society* 23, no. 5 (September 2003): 675–84, 682.

3. Edward F. McQuarrie, Jessica Miller, and Barbara J. Phillips, "The Megaphone Effect: Taste and Audience in Fashion Blogging," *Journal of Consumer Research* 40, no. 1 (June 2013): 136–58.

4. Harry R. Moody, "From Successful Aging to Conscious Aging," *Successful Aging through the Life Span: Intergenerational Issues in Health*, ed. May L. Wykle, Peter J. Whitehouse, and Diana L. Morris (New York: Springer, 2005), 55–68, 64.

5. Margaret Manning, "This Jamie Lee Curtis Quote about Aging Is Right on the Money," *Sixty and Me*, 2015, http://sixtyandme.com/jamie-lee-curtis-quote-about-aging/.

6. Nikolas Rose, *Inventing Our Selves: Psychology, Power, and Personhood* (Cambridge: Cambridge University Press, 1998), 154. Also see Richard Sennett, *The Culture of the New Capitalism* (New Haven, CT: Yale University Press, 2006). On the related notion of persons modeling themselves on the concept of a "brand," see Joseph E. Davis, "The Commodification of Self," *Hedgehog Review* 5, no. 2 (Summer 2003): 41–49.

7. According to political scientist Robert Crawford: "Health is not a given, nor is it simply a result of good luck or heredity, two frequently mentioned alternatives. Neither is it believed to be an outcome of normal life activities, such as one's work, upbringing or current lifestyle. Health must be achieved." See Crawford, "A Cultural Account of 'Health': Control, Release and the Social Body," in *Issues in the Political Economy of Health Care*, ed. John B. McKinlay (London: Tavistock, 1984), 60–103. On the role of the body to identity, see Bryan S. Turner, *The Body and Society*, 3rd ed. (Los Angeles: Sage, 2008). For an empirical study, see Peter Öberg and Lars Tornstam, "Youthfulness and Fitness—Identity Ideals for All Ages?," *Journal of Aging and Identity* 6, no. 1 (March 2001): 15–29.

8. John A. Vincent, "Ageing Contested: Anti-Ageing Science and the Cultural Construction of Old Age," *Sociology* 40, no. 4 (August 2006): 681–98, 689.

9. Margaret Manning, "Fashion for Women over 60—Look Fabulous without Trying to Look Younger," *Sixty and Me*, 2013, http://sixtyandme.com/fashion-after-60-how-to-look-fabulous-without-trying-to-look-younger/.

10. John W. Rowe and Robert L. Kahn, *Successful Aging* (New York: Pantheon Books, 1998).

11. "A good old age, in this definition," according to one critique, "is just an old age with minimum sickness or frailty, as much like youth or midlife as possible." See Moody, "From Successful Aging to Conscious Aging," 60.

12. Of course, the older you get, the more likely you are to fail. See studies in Peter Martin, Norene Kelly, Boaz Kahana, Eva Kahana, Bradley J. Willcox, D. Craig Willcox, and Leonard W. Poon, "Defining Successful Aging: A Tangible or Elusive Concept?," *The Gerontologist* 55, no. 1 (February 2015): 14–25, 18.

13. See, for example, Martha B. Holstein and Meredith Minkler, "Self, Society, and the 'New Gerontology,'" *The Gerontologist* 43, no. 6 (December 2003): 787–96.

14. Sarah Lamb, "Permanent Personhood or Meaningful Decline? Toward a Critical Anthropology of Successful Aging," *Journal of Aging Studies* 29, no. 1 (April 2014): 41–52.

15. Michael A. Flatt, Richard A. Settersten Jr., Roselle Ponsaran, and Jennifer R. Fishman, "Are 'Anti-Aging Medicine' and 'Successful Aging' Two Sides of the Same Coin? Views of Anti-Aging Practitioners," *Journals of Gerontology*, Series B: *Psychological Sciences and Social Sciences* 68, no. 6 (September 2013): 944–55.

16. Arlene Weintraub estimates the size of the antiaging industry at $88 billion. See Weintraub, *Selling the Fountain of Youth: How the Anti-Aging Industry Made a Disease Out of Getting Old—and Made Billions* (New York: Basic Books, 2010), 3.

17. Vincent, "Ageing Contested."

18. The Longevity and Stem Cell Centre of Houston, for example, notes that "with services such as Stem Cell Therapy, Hormone Replacement Therapy (for Menopause and Low Testosterone), Platelet Rich Plasma Therapy, Hyperbaric Oxygen Therapy, and more, we are able to mitigate the debilitating and disabling diseases associated with aging." From the center's homepage at http://longevitycentres.com.

19. See, for instance, Vincent, "Ageing Contested."

20. Mary Midgley, "Death and the Human Animal," *Philosophy Now* 89 (March/April 2012): 10–13.

21. In the words of Norbert Elias, "The dream of the elixir of life and of the fountain of youth is very ancient. But it is only in our day that it has taken on scientific, or pseudo-scientific, form." See Elias, *The Loneliness of the Dying* (New York: Continuum, 1985), 47. Further, see Bryan S. Turner, *Can We Live Forever? A Sociological and Moral Inquiry* (New York: Anthem Press, 2009), and Weintraub, *Selling the Fountain of Youth*.

22. Flatt et al., "Are 'Anti-Aging Medicine' and 'Successful Aging' Two Sides of the Same Coin?," 952.

23. Ivan Illich, *Medical Nemesis: The Expropriation of Health* (New York: Pantheon, 1976), 134.

24. Moody, "From Successful Aging to Conscious Aging," 60.

25. Joseph Lathrop, *The Infirmities and Comforts of Old Age* (Springfield, MA: Brewer, 1805), 4–6.

26. Elias, *The Loneliness of the Dying*, 2, 12, 40, 85.

27. Vivek Murthy, "Work and the Loneliness Epidemic," *Harvard Business Review*, October 12, 2017, https://hbr.org/cover-story/2017/09/work-and-the-loneliness-epidemic. The Caciappos offer this list of deleterious effects: "increased anxiety, hostility and social withdrawal; fragmented sleep and daytime fatigue; increased vascular resistance and altered gene expression and immunity; decreased impulse control; increased negativity and depressive symptoms; and increased age-related cognitive decline and risk of dementia." See John Cacioppo and Steph-

anie Cacioppo, "Loneliness Is a Modern Epidemic in Need of Treatment," *New Scientist*, December 30, 2014, https://www.newscientist.com/article/dn26739-loneliness-is-a-modern-epidemic-in-need-of-treatment#.VRKpX2TF9Cw.

28. Katie Hafner, "Researchers Confront an Epidemic of Loneliness," *New York Times*, September 5, 2016, https://www.nytimes.com/2016/09/06/health/lonliness-aging-health-effects.html.

29. Cacioppo and Cacioppo, "Loneliness Is a Modern Epidemic."

30. In a poignant article in the *Lancet*, the British physician Ishani Kar-Purkayastha describes her encounters in the hospital with an old woman who, though well, had no desire to return home, where she lived her days in isolation. She asks the doctor if she has a cure for loneliness. Kar-Purkayastha writes, "I wish I could prescribe her some antidepressants and be satisfied that I had done my best, but the truth is she's not clinically depressed. It's just that she has been left behind by a world that no longer revolves around her, not even the littlest bit of it." Ishani Kar-Purkayastha, "An Epidemic of Loneliness," *Lancet* 376, no. 9758 (December 2010): 2114–15, 2115.

31. Public policy responses predictably adopt aspects of the same medicalized perspective and orientation to loneliness as a problem to be solved. In January 2018, the British government made news when Prime Minister Theresa May announced her government's plans to "tackle loneliness." According to the official press release, May was appointing the Minister for Sport and Civil Society to take a ministerial "lead for loneliness," that would work with various stakeholders to "shine a light on the issue and pull together all strands of government to create the first ever strategy" and "end the acceptance of loneliness for good." In addition to "improved mental health support" and other "existing work," the "different initiatives" would include community efforts to reach out to lonely people, foster interaction, and "build more integrated and resilient communities." In her remarks, the minister for sport and civil society expressed the underlying assumption of loneliness as a type of medical condition that people suffer from and pledged to "make significant progress in defeating" it. Prime Minister's Office, "PM Commits to Government-Wide Drive to Tackle Loneliness," January 17, 2018, https://www.gov.uk/government/news/pm-commits-to-government-wide-drive-to-tackle-loneliness.

32. Quoted in Moody, "From Successful Aging to Conscious Aging," 55.

CHAPTER TWO

The Structural-Ethical Source of the Matter
The Medical-Industrial Complex

SHARON R. KAUFMAN

> *To be a medical citizen is to concern oneself both with the realm of politics and social justice and with clinical judgment. . . . We are in this sense all medical citizens, each one of us capable of using medicine as a way of thinking about society, and of society and politics as ways of understanding medical outcomes.*
> —Charles E. Rosenberg, *Our Present Complaint*

Treatments, technologies, and health policies have created immense challenges for everyone, those who work in medicine and those on the receiving end. I've been concerned with how each of these features of the medical landscape shapes the values and practices of clinical work, our personal sensibilities, and our national debates. In addition, medicine, as an institution, is influencing two other things: our collective experience of social obligation and our most intimate concerns about love and about how to express it.

Patients and all healthcare consumers are shaping medicine also. Our expectations and hopes about medical promise influence what happens in those drafty exam rooms when doctors and patients together talk about and decide what to do. We demand a lot from medicine, and we complain about it a lot, too. One could say that, as a society, both our demands and our complaints are at an all-time high.

Medicine's ability to prolong wanted life is a positive development. Yet the ability and desire to employ life-extending treatments now exists in an ever-aging society in which many older persons, their families, and their health providers face the quandary of whether those treatments bring with them too much pain and suffering. Where is the line between "enough" and "too much" treatment? I began to think about the quandary of that line, between enough and too much intervention, while I was conducting a study of hospitals and how death occurs there.

Most everyone claims to want to die at home, without tubes and machines. And although increasing numbers of patients are enrolled in hospice and palliative care, most of us still die in hospitals, and more than a quarter of those hospitalized still die after a prolonged stay in an intensive care unit there. Patients and families have been complaining for a long time that medicine does not attend to suffering or to wishes of the critically ill. Physicians, for their part, complain that patients and their families don't know when to stop, don't know when to say "no" to advanced technologies and procedures that do not restore health and may only prolong suffering.

The disquiet from both sides of the hospital bed remains ongoing, approximately twenty-five years after it began. I wanted to continue investigating why and how. So I began to pay closer attention to how hospital routines and complaints are anchored in other, more far-reaching social phenomena. For medicine is, of course, deeply embedded in the socioeconomic spheres of our society, spheres of influence that operate farther upstream, well before the very end of life. The successes of medicine, together with our expectations about it, are organizing, in new ways, how we think about health in advanced age and what "normal" aging should look like.

The demand for interventions, especially new ones, and the desire to fix everything now includes fixing our mortality. We certainly want to extend our own lives, but not past a certain point. The quandary has made the topic of control over the timing of death a national preoccupation.

In 2002 I began to observe older patients, those aged seventy and older, in specialty clinics where they were often offered life-prolonging therapies. I concentrated on cardiac devices, dialysis, kidney and liver transplantation, and cancer treatments. I listened to hundreds of patients, physicians, and family members deliberate about what to do. After scores of visits, I began to connect the conversations doctors and patients were having with each other to the bigger picture of institutions, politics, and economics. I started tracing the themes that emerged in clinic conversations about evidence and expectations, norms and standards, risks, hope and ambivalence, the urge to try everything, and the demand to stop. The talk mostly settled on scientific evidence, standards of care, risk reduction, and necessary treatments. And that talk led me to investigate how and why these phenomena have come to organize our "more is always better" approach to medicine. I started to focus on the larger engines of the biomedical economy, the research and insurance industries, and their impact on what we do when life is at stake.

What emerged was my realization that there is a hidden chain of connections among science, politics, industry, and insurance that organizes evidence-making and drives the US healthcare system. Hidden as well is the ethos that supports those connections and impacts governance.

That chain of drivers, those mostly unseen forces, have a powerful impact on what happens to us, what we agonize over, and what we decide to do about our own longevity and the lives of those we care about. I also began to understand how radically medicine has changed since we entered the new millennium. Several developments have coalesced in the past two decades, altering how medicine is practiced and therefore, on what doctors, patients, and families must deliberate. For example, there is more private industry involvement in all aspects of healthcare, from research to treatment; there are greater numbers of treatment options than ever before; and the United States is an aging society. Those over eighty-five are the fastest-growing cohort.

None of these developments is a secret. Yet, taken together, their effects on physicians' practices and patients' demands have been hidden from view. Together, they have created what I'm calling a *perfect storm* in healthcare.

I turn to a brief description of each phenomenon. The multibillion-dollar biomedical research engine, with its emphasis on the clinical trials enterprise, is where evidence-making begins. The infrastructure and high value of evidence-based medicine and clinical trials prioritize thinking about what constitutes responsible healthcare. Those phenomena are the dominant apparatuses of truth-making in medicine.

How do they work? Trial *findings* are converted into *best evidence for treatment*. And then that evidence generates treatment standards. This is how scientific innovation organizes physicians' work, healthcare finance, and patients' and families' expectations about what is normal and needed. The cultural capital of evidence-based medicine, clinical trials, and the standards they set create a unique quandary in contemporary medicine: when, where, and how to draw the line between too much and enough intervention. How should one live with the tools medicine offers?

Evidence-based medicine is itself complicated by three interrelated developments that permeate American life, that are inherent in the global biomedical economy, and that control the quandary of the line. These are, first, the increased role and influence of private industry. In 1980, thirty-two percent of clinical research was funded by private pharma, device, and biotech companies. Today, sixty-five percent of biomedical research is funded by private industry, whose goal is always to increase market share. Second, all those clinical trials have generated more evidence of therapeutic value and an ever-increasing number of standard treatment options. Third, our national priority on new technologies has influenced our collective perspective on the timing of death. Today, in the United States, most deaths, regardless of a person's age, have come to be considered premature.

All of the outcome studies, practice guidelines, and teaching tools within the vast evidence-based medicine matrix have a single goal: to provide a stronger scientific foundation for clinical practice. Yet that scientifically based (and especially numerically based) matrix omits the social, non-scientific, and messy features of healthcare delivery that influence what doctors do and what happens to patients.

Consider the following five, decidedly non-scientific, features of clinical medicine: (1) Physicians sometimes act against their own best judgment and recommend or prescribe interventions despite their known lack of efficacy. (2) Patients and families ask for treatments that have not been proven to show benefit in studies, and physicians, not infrequently, acquiesce to their requests. (3) Industry is slow to remove from the marketplace drugs and devices that lack benefit (or that prove to be harmful), and doctors may be slow to refuse to use them. (4) Once a treatment is reimbursed by Medicare, the dynamics of hospital and medical center economics and physician prescribing patterns make it nearly impossible for all concerned to say "no" to it. Medicare reimbursement thus shapes standard-making and ethical necessity. It becomes the ethics of managing life. (5) Whether treatments that benefit some carefully selected trial participants will also benefit a more diverse group of patients, especially children and older persons, is always a question, and often a troubling one for doctors.

As devices such as automatic implantable cardioverter defibrillators (ICDs) become smaller and as techniques for implanting them become safer, physicians and the public have learned to view them as standard interventions that one does not easily refuse. In the United States, these developments produce a sense that life extension is open-ended as long as one treats risk. That is the prevailing, ordinary logic that drives so much treatment. But when do we stop treating risks?

The ICD was used sparingly until 2002 for those who had already survived a potentially lethal heart attack and were at high risk of another life-threatening cardiac event. Then its use began to rise substantially. Why? Nine clinical trials of ICD use were conducted between 2002 and 2005, each one showing varying degrees of benefit among patient populations that had not experienced a potentially life-threatening heart rhythm. Taken together, the findings from those nine trials provided increasing *evidence of benefit* of the ICD for survival, and that evidence led Medicare, in 2005, to expand the eligibility criteria for reimbursement to include primary prevention for those who have never suffered a potentially fatal cardiac rhythm. The floodgates opened.

Now these devices have become the standard of care for patients with moderate to severe heart disease. The important thing about the ICD is that, in treating a potentially lethal arrhythmia, it prevents sudden death (the silent heart attack in the night), the kind of death many say they actually want in late life. Yet the device is difficult to refuse, even very late in life. Why? Because evidence organizes its expanded use and because it seems to go against medical progress and common sense to say "no" to it. It has become an ordinary part of the medico-socioethical landscape. The effects of this logic most affect the oldest patients.

There is no question of the unequivocal value of this device for preventing young people from dying. Yet today, more than 110,000 patients in the United States receive ICDs each year. Most persons with ICDs are older and sicker, with underlying cardiac disease, and the electrical shocks from an ICD do not necessarily extend an older person's life or improve its quality. Indeed, the ICD transforms the immediate risk of death into the near certainty of progressive heart failure. The hope of this life-extending treatment comes up against a prolonged, unwanted kind of late life and dying.

Older patients and their families must ponder an individual ethic of life extension. For patients, it often goes like this: Given my current age—that is, how long I have already lived—how much longer do I want to try to live, given what the clinic offers?

Consider Sam Tolleson (a pseudonym), who, like some other patients with ICDs, endured the pain of the device's shocks and the knowledge that his debility was being prolonged. At age eighty-eight, Sam had been living with cardiac disease for twenty-five years by the time I met him. Tall and thin with piercing blue eyes and a shock of thick white hair, he used oxygen and walked slowly, bent over his walker. He graciously welcomed me to sit down in his apartment and chat. Following a second heart attack at age eighty, he awoke in the hospital and was told that physicians had implanted a pacemaker that included a defibrillator. The physicians were following standard practice, doing what was appropriate both to stabilize his heart rate (via the pacemaker) and prevent sudden death from a future heart attack (via the ICD). Mr. Tolleson noted that it wasn't until sometime after getting the defibrillator that he learned what it would do.

About two years before we met, when he was eighty-six, the ICD had begun to shock his potentially lethal cardiac rhythms back to normal. Over a period of several months, Mr. Tolleson was shocked fifteen times. "There is no question," he offered, "that those shocks extended my life. It's very likely that one of those episodes, without the defibrillator, would have been my last." The first ten shocks were, he reported, "spread out, over weeks." But when he received five shocks in one day, he decided that he had had enough. "They were more and more painful. The very thought that I was going to have another one, I couldn't take it."

So he made an appointment to have the defibrillator part of the device turned off. This choice is highly unusual. It simply does not occur to most patients or their families that the device, once placed under the skin, can easily be deactivated and that patients can make that choice. Studies have shown that most physicians never discuss that possibility with patients. Mr. Tolleson noted, "Both the doctor and the technician [from the device company] were reluctant to turn it off. But I convinced them . . . and that distressed my family too. The family was very upset with me. I have three children, and they all cried. I had to talk with them about it, and I felt terrible after I talked with them." He continued, "Perhaps I should just have done what they wanted me to do: keep the ICD. But life is getting harder all the time."

Mr. Tolleson died two days after our conversation.

How can we think about his decision and its context? Scientific evidence, routine reimbursement, standards of care, specialists' expertise, industry's goal to sell devices, and medicine's mandate to extend life are all strong forces. Mr. Tolleson found himself needing to defend his decision to turn off the defibrillator—both to his family and to the medical staff. He had crossed the line he did not wish to cross.

Since increasing numbers of those on the receiving end of ICDs are now well over eighty, the device is reshaping the aging experience and the dying transition for significant numbers of people. It staves off death but does not improve health. It turns life-threatening disease into a chronic condition, enabling people to grow older in need of more intervention, more risk awareness, and more prevention—all at the same time. This is where evidence has come to rest in the case of the ICD—in the kind of death we are asked to choose and in a new, uncomfortable engagement with our own role in the timing of death.

These are widespread preoccupations now for millions of patients (and not only those with ICDs), illustrating how ethics has been offloaded onto patients and their families. Ordinary medicine entangles patients and families in a new obligation to increase longevity because they experience the balancing act, that weighing of the worth of more life against the worth of more treatment, that judgment about crossing the line. Physicians are not always aware of these sensibilities.

Physicians have dilemmas about the ICD as well, especially with the idea that the risk of sudden death is a scientific reason for employing the device. One physician who implants ICDs spoke for others when he reported:

> It becomes very controversial sometimes, and that's one of the sources of my personal unrest. It's very tricky to sit down with an eighty-eight-year-old patient or their loving family—and by now they've heard about this technology—and to say, "You know, he does meet the clinical criteria, but really, at his age, it may not be the right thing. If he were to have a dangerous arrhythmia—that's the way people pass quietly in their sleep. That may be a natural moment at the end of the person's life. Sudden death is actually a pretty good way to go.

Make no mistake; this technology extends wanted life for many people. That is the crux of the matter. It has also opened up an ever-expanding market for other cardiac devices, because when this one no longer does the job, one can graduate to the left ventricular assist device (LVAD), or heart pump, which costs ten times as much. Each device triggers quandaries about how one can or should live in relation to medical treatment, especially as one ages. Nowhere do I seek to make a case for or against the use of the ICD or any other therapy. Rather, the issue for me is how clinical norms and our very lives have been caught up in the perfect storm of ordinary, evidence-based medicine. How and why evidence-based therapeutics bring increasing numbers of patients and families, our politicians, and indeed our entire society, to face the quandary of the line and to complain loudly about the systems that create that line. As more of us come to want, need, or acquiesce to these treatments, how do the profound effects of evidence on medical practice and everyday life organize what I have called our postprogress predicament?

Note

This chapter is adapted from my book *Ordinary Medicine: Extraordinary Treatments, Longer Lives, and Where to Draw the Line* (Durham, NC: Duke University Press, 2015).

CHAPTER THREE

Beyond Avoidance and Autonomy

PAUL SCHERZ

Contemporary ethics has a difficult time addressing the topics of aging and death, difficulties that reflect the broader cultural problems discussed in the previous chapter. Ethicists tend to favor one of two strategies: to either avoid speaking about these concerns or advocate for patient autonomy in relation to them. This latter strategy, I will argue, is merely another method of avoidance. It is not surprising that contemporary ethics has problems with such issues, since these same difficulties are found in the major sources that ethicists draw upon. For example, the utilitarianism that guides much of our daily existence and policy decision-making argues that pleasure or the satisfaction of interests is good and pain or the frustration of one's desires is bad. Since no one desires to grow old and have the problems to which the aging body is prone, aging becomes something to be avoided. Death is even worse, ruling out all satisfaction of desire. Because of these difficulties, consequentialist ethicists ignore the topic for the most part. Alternatively, many of the consequentialist ethicists who do address these problems argue that we might avoid them by ending aging or extending life indefinitely.[1]

One might think that Aristotle, the most common source for today's virtue ethicists, would serve as a counterweight to such consequentialist claims, as he does in so many other instances. Yet even Aristotle is not much help on aging and death. Unlike most other ancient philosophers, he does not talk much about death, and, when he does, it is generally only in regard to technical issues, like delineating the virtue of courage.[2] He is even less helpful for finding productive ways to think about aging, since his discussion is almost completely negative. He describes elderly men as timid, cynical, small-minded, cowardly, not generous, and too fond of themselves![3] It does not seem, in his writings, like a stage of life given to virtue or flourishing.

Things get a little better when one turns to liberal deontological ethics. This descendant of Kantianism prizes autonomy, the ability to make one's own moral decisions, and, above all else, respecting persons as ends in themselves. Thus, this ethic moves in a proceduralist direction, creating rules so that everyone can make their own decisions as to how to confront the various problems of aging and end-of-life care. As I will discuss below, this proceduralist focus on autonomy has become the central theme of bioethics.[4] Such an ethic might make room for more productive conversations on aging and death. Yet this ethic also has its problems, since the challenge that we are facing is that people do not actually know how they ought, as individuals, to face aging and death.[5] Our society lacks the cultural resources provided by older traditions that would allow individuals to confront decline and death within a meaningful framework. In the absence of such traditions, individuals are forced to improvise at the most vulnerable moments of their lives, when powerful forces and cultural factors push people to fear aging and death and thus avoid them at all costs. Further, despite the formal autonomy individuals have in decision-making, structural factors in the delivery of medicine, discussed by Sharon Kaufman, push patients to receive ever more complicated, burdensome, and expensive care.[6] Even when autonomy enables a patient to assert himself against these factors, its centrality sometimes carries with it a distinctive vision of the good life, a vision of a detached independence, which itself avoids a central aspect of aging that I will discuss in this chapter in detail, namely dependency. Thus a more adequate and substantive ethic is needed to provide people with the resources to confront aging and death in medical decision-making as well as in their daily lives.

In this chapter I will first examine how these tendencies toward avoidance or autonomy play out in many of the problems of contemporary bioethics. In the second part of the chapter, I will then point to two elements that might serve as foundations for a more adequate ethic of aging. More specifically, I hope to pick out common threads describing persons in the face of aging and death that are emerging from religious ethics, philosophy, and social science. These aspects might serve as a point of contact or conversation among those who do not merely want to avoid aging or assert autonomy in the face of decline.

In this constructive portion of the chapter I will focus on developments in the ethics of character. A character or virtue-based ethics looks less at the casuistry of specific actions, although it does address those, but instead seeks to determine what kinds of dispositions one must have to live well and how one should relate to others in order to live flourishing lives in community. The ethics of character discussed here draws on movements in philosophy that are developing strands of ancient ethics like Stoicism that differ from Aristotle, philosophical schools that were also widely drawn on by diverse religious traditions such as Christianity, Islam, and Judaism.[7] Further, an ethics of character allows for conversation with movements in the social sciences like the anthropology of ethics.[8] These insights can help us to develop a richer picture of the human, a better philosophical anthropology that can move beyond the autonomy/avoidance dichotomy.

Bioethics and Autonomy at the End of Life

Before beginning that constructive portion of the argument, though, it is important to understand how bioethics is currently addressing aging and death. Contemporary bioethics predominantly follows a system called principlism. It posits four principles that should guide medical decision-making: autonomy, beneficence, nonmaleficence, and justice.[9] As many critics have noted, in practice, in most cases these principles reduce to autonomy: beneficence and nonmaleficence are generally taken to mean fostering or not harming what one autonomously decides are one's interests (although there are exceptional cases involving incompetent patients). There have been some salutary movements to take justice more into account in the form of attempting to ensure the provision of care to those who have been denied it in the past due to poverty or discrimination, but, as Sharon Kaufman discusses in chapter 2, the push to provide more care at the end of life is not always an innocent development. There have also been some justice-based calls to cap end-of-life care in order to secure the common good of public finances, but those have largely been rejected in theory and practice in favor of autonomous decision-making in regard to care.

This focus on autonomy at the end of life led to some of bioethics' early triumphs. In 1977, Karen Ann Quinlan, a young woman in a persistent vegetative state, was trapped by the growing medical-technological push to avoid death at all cost.[10] Doctors were unwilling to remove her from her ventilator because such a withdrawal of care seemed tantamount to murder. It took the courts to uphold her family's ability to decide about her fate. An even more troubling evasion in those days was the lack of honesty in relation to terminal illness. Doctors feared telling patients when they were dying because such news might drive patients into despair.[11] Because of this, many patients were unable to prepare for death and, in the many cases when other family members knew what the patient did not, it resulted in strained relationships and a last few weeks of life clouded by secrets. A focus on honesty and autonomy has forced medical staff to speak truthfully about terminal illnesses. Of course medical conversations about death are still shrouded in evasions, but at least doctors can no longer straightforwardly lie about a terminal condition or deny the removal of a ventilator from a terminal patient.

Thus much good came from this push for autonomy, especially as it confronted our culture's avoidance of death. Yet, taken as a lone or even the main ethical principle, autonomy is a radically deficient way to think about aging. The centrality of autonomy arises from a modern Western vision of the person.[12] In this understanding, the person is an independent director of her life, standing detached in many ways from the bonds of community, tradition, external circumstances, or relationships. One may choose to make these things important, but they are not constitutive of the person in this vision. The problem is that little in this image of the person reflect the reality of aging and death. Both happen whether one wills them or not, and generally against one's will. Far from a time of independent action, they reveal one's dependence on others. In the face of these phenomena, the buffers fall away from the self, revealing one's neediness for relationship and one's vulnerability to external events. Autonomy cannot answer the issues of old age, and solutions based on it will lead to problematic results.

One can see how this autonomous ideal fails to connect to the reality of aging and dying in one of the greatest disappointments of early bioethics. Beginning in earnest in the 1970s, many ethicists who focused on end-of-life ethics argued for living wills, what we today would call advance directives.[13] These documents allow an individual to specify what kind of care they should receive in the event that they become incompetent—whether they should be kept on a ventilator, how long they should continue in intensive care if they enter a coma, etc. Such a document would allow the patient autonomy through her surrogates even when she could no longer exercise it herself. In 1990 the new Patient Self-Determination Act required medical facilities to inform all patients of their right to execute such documents. Great hopes were raised. However, by 2005 the President's Council on Bioethics joined most other voices in bioethics in concluding that these documents were failures. First, their architects failed to understand the difficulty of fully specifying one's wishes, leaving much to be decided by the surrogate. Individuals fail to foresee situations, and many have a poor grasp of what a medical or life situation might be like when it actually occurs.[14] Many people mistake how they will emotionally respond to a crisis situation, reflecting findings from behavioral psychology that indicate that people are poor judges of their future states.[15] For example, in many cases people fill out forms indicating they do not want any extraordinary care, but then when faced with a choice, choose invasive care options, leaving families confused as to how to move ahead in the future once the patient is no longer competent.[16] Further, families sometimes disagree over interpretation, and ethicists failed to realize how much even such an exercise of autonomy was dependent on one's relationships with others. Probably the biggest difficulty with them, however, is that people are unwilling to actually fill them out, and even when they do fill them out are unwilling to think long and hard about death. In my experience, people want these conversations to be over with quickly, thus short-circuiting the long, difficult discussions of different options and possibilities necessary to give a surrogate a true idea of what a person would like in situations of death and disability. People want to avoid the conversation about death, and you cannot force someone to be autonomous.

Even more concerted attempts to move beyond overtreatment at the end of life reveal a failure to take aging and decline seriously. Michael Banner gives two examples of the failure of the frameworks currently employed by society in relation to aging: assisted suicide and hospice care.[17] These models of confronting death depend on an inadequate narrative of independent agency as well as an overemphasis on acute terminal conditions such as cancer. In reality, the problem that most contemporary people face is what Banner has called the long dying of late modernity: long periods of gradual decline, frailty, and disability; chronic disease requiring repeated hospitalizations; slowly developing dementias; and the concomitant segregation of the elderly into specialized facilities.

With regard to assisted suicide, current legalization efforts are ostensibly aimed at acute, generally painful terminal diseases like cancer, requiring a prognosis of death within six months. Yet if one looks to the few studies on the topic, many of the common reasons people give for desiring suicide are not related to pain, which almost always can be ameliorated, but with things like the loss of self-sufficiency or becoming a burden on others.[18] In its framing in bioethics and mainstream culture, assisted suicide goes along with the desire to be the detached, autonomous self of the modern West.[19] Once self-sufficiency is lost and one becomes dependent, it seems as if one's dignity and reasons for living are lost. Many disability rights advocates fear the expansion of assisted suicide and euthanasia because these are not concerns limited to acute terminal illness. Indeed, loss of self-sufficiency and feeling like a burden to others are part of many aspects of the human condition, such as disability and especially the physical and mental decline frequently experienced in old age. Other countries, such as Belgium and the Netherlands, have already seen the expansion of assisted suicide to other categories, such as depression, and many bioethicists argue for such an expansion in the United States.[20]

Somewhat surprisingly, hospice care, which serves as a radically alternative framework to that of assisted suicide, is also constrained by the framing in terms of autonomy and acute care, according to Banner. The hospice movement sprang from the universally praised work of Dame Cicely Saunders, who advocated the provision of a setting in which people can receive holistic end-of-life care, including medical palliation alongside spiritual preparation for death. Like most such movements, its character has changed as it has spread. There are now many criticisms of hospice care: it has become too corporate; it has moved from a rich embedded spirituality to generic spiritual care driven by counseling; and, rather than providing sensitive, careful palliative care, it just sedates people until death.[21] The concerns that Banner raises are that, first, it serves only a subset of patients with acute illness, since Medicare funds hospice care only if the patient has a life expectancy of six months or less. Indeed, Cardinal John O'Connor reported receiving threats from insurance companies to cease funding his diocese's hospice center for cancer patients because it was keeping its patients alive too long.[22] Thus, the framework of hospice care also fails to address the long decline frequently seen in contemporary aging. Second, hospice care, too, is primarily about taking autonomous control over one's death. In this sense, it is about both gaining spiritual control and prizing control away from doctors. Banner is concerned that this focus on autonomy does not deal well with those in states of dependency and mental decline.

Thus we are in a situation in which bioethics lacks the effective means of addressing the primary problems facing our society in terms of old age. Bioethics has primarily focused on autonomy, which is an important aspect of being human but does not provide the best lens for addressing these issues. Its picture of the evening of life has become narrowed—focused on control over the decisions surrounding death, especially as death occurs in the setting of high-technology medicine in response to acute terminal illness. Because of this focus, the ethical concerns surrounding aging have largely dropped out of the picture of mainstream bioethics. Moreover, essential aspects of aging and dying, like the role of family and other relations, increasing dependency, and fears of burdening others, go unaddressed. Finally, a focus on autonomy has failed to overcome the cultural momentum to avoid death because the patients who have been granted the authority to choose autonomously still largely avoid looking death in the face until it has become too late to do anything other than abandon oneself to technological medicine or isolation in specialized care facilities.

Human Dependency

In such a situation, where our current ethical resources fail us, it seems right to look elsewhere for the tools that are needed to better address aging and dying. These alternative resources could come from other cultures, from other historical eras, or from aspects of living traditions that still exist in our own society. In all of these places, one finds very different ways of approaching aging and dying from those found in contemporary ethics. Moreover, they paint very different pictures of what it means to be human than does the dominant autonomy-focused anthropology. Many of these alternative hermeneutics highlight two very distinct aspects of the human prefigured in the first part of the chapter that I will explore in more detail in the rest of the chapter. The first is that dependency and vulnerability are central aspects of the human condition. The second is that meditation on death shapes life in a positive way.

In one of his later books, Alasdair MacIntyre argued that the traditional Western definition of humans as rational animals was incomplete.[23] Instead, humans should be termed "dependent rational animals." This term is not meant to depreciate rationality, the most morally salient aspect of which is our ability to reason about and freely choose courses of action. Humans are still autonomous creatures by nature. What it does do is highlight that humans are also embodied creatures made to live in community with others. Humans are dependent because one cannot generate all the things that one needs to live, or especially to live well, on one's own. Humans depend on a community of others in order to flourish. Humans are dependent because of the way the life course of creatures like us is structured. Children enter the world completely vulnerable, dependent on the care of others, and at the end of life one's physical frailties again leave one dependent upon families and communities for care. Humans are dependent because we are embodied beings, instantiated in the ever-changing, ever-imperfect material world. This material embodiment makes one continually vulnerable—vulnerable to injury, to disease, to pain, and to disabilities of all sorts. These vulnerabilities have the potential to leave one dependent on others for both practical care and emotional support while undergoing suffering. Finally, humans are dependent because we are not the authors of our own being; we did not bring the world around us into existence. Commentators have discussed this aspect of human dependency in terms of the giftedness of life or wonder at the fact of being.[24] Humans are dependent on genetic, social, and structural factors even for who one is, and one lies vulnerable to the changing circumstances of the world around us. Christian commentators talk about this aspect of human existence as the fact that we are creatures, that we are created, not in the sense of denying evolution but in the sense that the entire world depends for its being on a source that lies outside itself. Rather than take this lack of control as a matter engendering fear, it can be a source for wonder and joy.

If one takes dependency as central to what it is to be human, two corollaries emerge. First, care for the dependent becomes important. To begin with, it is a responsibility emerging from the most basic ethical injunction, the Golden Rule. Just as we all were children, we are all susceptible to diseases, and many of us will succumb to the frailties of old age, we therefore ought to care for those currently in those states as we would wish to be cared for ourselves. Thus Judaism and Christianity make the care of the widow and orphan a cornerstone of the ethical evaluation of any society. The rejection of these vulnerable classes calls down condemnation on a society. Moreover, this care is not only a duty but also a part of a flourishing human life, a way to develop in virtue as well as to develop a rich pattern of relationships. This is one of the key insights to emerge from the development of a feminist ethics of care.[25]

A second corollary of this engagement with dependency is that none of the things that come along with the nature of humans as dependent rational animals should be considered shameful. As Cicero has Cato the Elder say in *De Senectute*, for the virtuous, "nothing which comes in the course of nature can seem evil."[26] Suffering, weakness, incontinence, or neediness are certainly unpleasant, but they arise from our nature as embodied beings, and thus should not be considered as experiences that degrade one's dignity. It is human to go through such experiences. The virtue of patience is oriented exactly toward enabling a person to deal with these vulnerabilities well. It is the current dominant picture of the person as detached and controlling his body and environment that leads one to reject these experiences of need and dependence as degrading. An overemphasis on autonomy causes us to mistake what it means to be human.

For Islam, Judaism, and Christianity, the humility that recognizes one's dependence on God is an attitude that ought to be fostered. For example, Saba Mahmood describes how women in Egypt's Islamic piety movement use embodied devotional practice to bring this pious subjectivity into being, even performing imaginative exercises to bring about the tears that are the sign of humility in prayer.[27] Christianity can also serve as a case study for how an understanding of humility, dependence, and vulnerability helps one to confront these problems. In Christianity, humility assumes a central role as the first step toward God and the foundation of the spiritual life. Pride, on the other hand, is the primordial sin because it refuses to recognize dependence on God and one's need for others. It rejects the relationality central to human existence. As one depends on God, one should serve others in their time of need.

It may seem that all of this focus on dependency and vulnerability sets humans in a bad light. Many have accused Christians of denigrating human embodiment precisely because of its emphasis on humility, dependency, and suffering. But in fact, dependence and humility become the route of exaltation through the figure of Christ. The key term is "kenosis," which means emptying and comes from Paul's letter to the Philippians, discussing how Jesus, "who, though he was in the form of God, did not regard equality with God something to be grasped. Rather, he emptied himself, taking the form of a slave, coming in human likeness; and found human in appearance, he humbled himself."[28] The second person of the Trinity humbled himself by taking on human nature in the Incarnation, with all the failings, weaknesses, vulnerabilities, and dependencies that that nature possesses. This humility, this self-emptying and setting aside of the forms of divine power, assimilates human nature to a divine Person. Further, Christ's humility is tied to the exaltation of the Resurrection.[29]

This notion of kenosis has become central in some discussions of aging and suffering in Christian ethics.[30] While Christian ethicists support medical and personal efforts to retain bodily functioning throughout the aging process, they recognize that, at some point, physical and mental decline will set in. At some point, the aging person will exchange the powerful, controlling form of human life found in one's prime for a form of weakness. One could try to deny this change as long as possible, seek routes to escape it in anti-aging technologies or life extension, become ashamed of it, or isolate oneself from others so that they will not witness this seeming humiliation. These are all evasions that will eventually fail. Instead, these theologians argue that as decline overtakes a person, she should actively assimilate the experience as a form of kenosis, transforming her understanding of what is occurring. It is not the voluntary kenosis of Christ, since it is involuntary in us. But, by not pridefully rejecting it, by instead humbly engaging it, we can imitate Christ, conforming ourselves to his example. God's power shines through and can become perfect in our weakness. It is through this humble imitation that every person can become exalted in Christ.

In Catholic spirituality, this engagement with suffering, vulnerability, and weakness can become an even more intimate participation in Christ's suffering on the Cross. Through this means the suffering of decline and weakness is united with what Christians see as the central event of history and becomes an opportunity to participate in the salvific work of that act. This doctrine is drawn from Paul, who says, "Now I rejoice in my sufferings for your sake, and in my flesh I am filling up what is lacking in the afflictions of Christ on behalf of his body, which is the church."[31] Recent papal writings have repeatedly referred to the seemingly antiquated practice of "offering up" one's suffering for others as central to affirming the nonindividualistic, relational anthropology of Catholicism.[32] John Paul II, who gave a powerful witness to Catholic doctrine on suffering and aging in his very public decline due to Parkinson's disease, referred to the communion of suffering Christians as "a multiple subject of [Christ's] supernatural power."[33] Through one's relationship with God, one's dependency, vulnerability, and weakness are paradoxically transformed into a source of agency and aid for the rest of the community, and the dependent becomes the one to whom the Church turns for spiritual aid. In this way, the sense of the uselessness and burdensomeness of the suffering, dependent person is obviated, as her spiritual work serves as an essential service for the salvation of others in the community.[34] Thus an understanding of humans as dependent, vulnerable, and relational can be essential for recovering a different understanding of the decline frequently present in aging. It is an agency that is not autonomous. Christianity offers one example of how such an alternative anthropology can function, but many other traditions can also serve to teach us better ways forward.

The Meditation on Death

In Christianity, Christ's death on the Cross is central to this model of kenosis, which leads to a second point: one needs to meditate on death in order to lead a good life. Thought on death certainly shapes a Christian life: Death serves as a transition to eternal life, sin is connected to death, baptism is understood as a participation in death, and life as a whole can be understood as an ongoing death to the self in order to live in Christ. Indeed, Michael Banner has suggested this last teaching as a possible Christian interpretation of gradual mental decline and dementia. Many have popularly understood it as a death before death. There are many problems with this language surrounding Alzheimer's, as Janelle Taylor argues in her beautiful piece on this issue and as advocates for those with dementia affirm.[35] But Banner wonders whether Christianity can positively reappropriate it as another painful step in the continuing duty to die to oneself in baptism. He asks, "Might we even come to speak of the possibility for those diagnosed with Alzheimer's of accepting the path before them as a vocation, as the saints accepted martyrdom—that is, as accepting in the death of the self which they face, a second baptism?"[36] This suggestive hint points to the possibilities of more forthrightly reappropriating Christian thought on death rather than avoiding the topic.

An encouragement to face death throughout life is not just a Christian trope, though. Robert Desjarlais has offered another example of the role that thought on death can play in a religious tradition in his discussion of the Hyolmo people of Nepal, whose form of Buddhism encourages much attention and training for death throughout life. It is a beautiful book investigating all aspects of death and mourning, but the most important aspect of the book for this argument is a short section on preparation for death. Dying well is important, since it is through dying well that one is able to release one's attachments to the body. "A dying self endeavors to dissolve the self";[37] thus it is a very different aim undertaken in death than in Christianity. Still, one's actions throughout life can shape whether one dies well or not, first through the karmic repayment of bad actions in this life or a previous one, but also, more importantly for this chapter, because being prepared to die well requires adequate training throughout life. Desjarlais notes that "many learn how to die. They undertake an apprenticeship on the subject, lest they approach it in an uninformed way and disturb their chances for a good rebirth."[38] If one does not think about one's death, one will "blunder through life in a foolish way." This thinking on death begins in childhood, when children play at death. Here one sees that reflection on dying plays an important role in life as a whole, shaping action and character.

One even need not be tied to a specific religious tradition to see the importance of reflection on death. While much of current philosophical ethics avoids questions of death and decline, these were central to older strands of Western philosophy. For Plato, Cicero, Montaigne, and many others, to practice philosophy was to learn how to die, because engaging with death was a central part of living a good life. Even in the last century, Heidegger thought that coming to terms with one's mortality is essential to living authentically.[39] Pierre Hadot provides perhaps the best examination of why this engagement with death is so important in his exploration of Hellenistic ethics, especially Stoicism.[40] Stoics undertook a number of philosophical practices in order to shape their character in line with their philosophical outlook. One of the most important of these was the *praemeditatio futurorum malorum*, the meditation on possible future evils and disasters.[41] The most important of these meditations was the *memento mori*, remembering that one and one's loved ones are mortal. In part, one thinks of the possibility of death so one will not be shocked and overcome by it when it hits. But, more importantly, meditating on death and other evils that may afflict a person shapes her life. It helps her to put things in their proper perspective, to not put too much importance on ambitions, slights, or material goods, since all will eventually be lost in death. It encourages a person to prepare herself morally and practically so that she will be ready for death. It helps a person to focus on the present moment rather than distracting himself with possible future plans, since he knows that his time is limited. It encourages a person to enjoy what she has, especially the presence of loved ones, since she has them for only a little time. As I have argued elsewhere, the misconception that we have an infinite future leads to our current distraction and focus on lesser goods.[42]

These Stoic practices of the self in relation to death were influential in the Christian *ars moriendi* tradition.[43] In the early fifteenth century, in the wake of the Black Death and the attendant broad focus on death in society, the Catholic Church developed a set of manuals to assist people at the deathbed and in preparation for death.[44] These manuals on the art of dying became enormously popular, inspiring a whole genre of books written by some of the best scholars of the day, such as Erasmus and Robert Bellarmine. These books were popular among many of the different Christian confessions, and they retained their popularity until the nineteenth century.

Part of the focus of these manuals was on the deathbed itself, providing detailed discussions on the temptations that the dying person might face, the prayers that should be said, and the importance of engaging the Christian sacraments. Yet, beginning with Erasmus's important intervention on the art of dying, these books also began to look at the relationship of dying well to how one lived one's life as a whole.[45] The idea was that to die well, one must first live well.[46] Living well entailed using one's life to prepare for death. One prepares for death throughout life by developing certain virtues, like courage. One must especially develop dispositions that will help him to accept death, such as a certain distance from worldly goods that will be lost in death, like wealth, ambition, or power.[47] If a person wishes to die well, he must also develop an acceptance of the will of God, thus emphasizing the importance of the humility discussed in the last section.[48] It is important to note that these virtues and dispositions are valuable not only at the deathbed; they are the sort of virtues that help one to deal with all of the difficulties and sufferings of daily life. The art of developing these virtues expanded preparation for death to the entirety of life, encouraging reflection and alteration of character so that one could both live and die better. This art in Christianity, in Buddhism, and ancient philosophy aimed to prepare one for a death that achieved ends that existed beyond this world, but all of these have important effects in this life as well.

All of these approaches encourage individuals to substantively confront the issue of aging and dying in a very different way than is found in mainstream contemporary ethics. By largely avoiding this topic, ethics loses the positive potential that a meditation on death can have both in helping us to prepare for the vicissitudes of aging and death and also in shaping us to live more flourishing lives in the present. By nurturing fantasies that we can escape death and decline, contemporary ethics, encouraged by contemporary culture, causes us to miss the positive potential that can be found in human weakness, leading to denial of the value of those suffering around us. Moreover, it leads us to mistake what it means to be human. The attempt to attain control over our dying through the exercise of autonomy clearly fails to properly recognize what we are as dependent, relational creatures. It is thus essential that we come to a better understanding of ourselves as mortal beings. We must learn to number our days, so that we may gain wisdom.[49]

Notes

1. See, for example, John Harris, *Enhancing Evolution: The Ethical Case for Making Better People* (Princeton, NJ: Princeton University Press, 2007).

2. Aristotle, *Nicomachean Ethics*, trans. Terence Irwin, 2nd ed. (Indianapolis: Hackett, 1999), III.6.

3. Aristotle, *Rhetoric*, II.13. Cited in Frits de Lange, *Loving Later Life: An Ethics of Aging* (Grand Rapids, MI: Eerdmans, 2015), 18.

4. See, for example, the discipline's most influential textbook, Tom L. Beauchamp and James F. Childress, *Principles of Biomedical Ethics*, 7th ed. (New York: Oxford University Press, 2012).

5. Allen Verhey, *The Christian Art of Dying: Learning from Jesus* (Grand Rapids: Eerdmans, 2011), 48–49.

6. Sharon R. Kaufman, *Ordinary Medicine: Extraordinary Treatments, Longer Lives, and Where to Draw the Line* (Durham, NC: Duke University Press Books, 2015).

7. For overviews of Hellenistic ethics, see Julia Annas, *The Morality of Happiness* (New York: Oxford University Press, 1993); Pierre Hadot, *Philosophy as a Way of Life: Spiritual Exercises from Socrates to Foucault*, trans. Arnold I. Davidson (Cambridge, MA: Blackwell, 1995); Martha Nussbaum, *The Therapy of Desire: Theory and Practice in Hellenistic Ethics* (Princeton, NJ: Princeton University Press, 1996); Michel Foucault, *The Hermeneutics of the Subject: Lectures at the Collège de France, 1981–82*, trans. Graham Burchell (New York: Palgrave Macmillan, 2005).

8. Important examples of the anthropology of ethics include Saba Mahmood, *Politics of Piety: The Islamic Revival and the Feminist Subject*, 2nd rev. ed. (Princeton, NJ: Princeton University Press, 2005); Joel Robbins, *Becoming Sin-*

ners: Christianity and Moral Torment in a Papua New Guinea Society (Berkeley, CA: University of California Press, 2004); Jarrett Zigon, *"HIV Is God's Blessing": Rehabilitating Morality in Neoliberal Russia* (Berkeley: University of California Press, 2010); James Laidlaw, *The Subject of Virtue: An Anthropology of Ethics and Freedom* (New York: Cambridge University Press, 2014); China Scherz, *Having People, Having Heart* (Chicago: University of Chicago Press, 2014).

9. These principles emerged out of the discussion leading to the Belmont Report on the ethics of human subjects research, but they are most fully developed in Beauchamp and Childress, *Principles of Biomedical Ethics*.

10. Albert Jonsen, *The Birth of Bioethics* (New York: Oxford University Press, 2003), 254–55.

11. For historical origins of this belief, see Shai Lavi, *The Modern Art of Dying: A History of Euthanasia in the United States* (Princeton, NJ: Princeton University Press, 2005), 54–57.

12. For history, analysis, and critique of this vision, see Charles Taylor, *Sources of the Self: The Making of the Modern Identity* (Cambridge: Cambridge University Press, 1992).

13. For the history and problems of these documents, see President's Council on Bioethics, *Taking Care: Ethical Caregiving in Our Aging Society* (Washington, DC: President's Council on Bioethics, 2005), 53–91.

14. The most famous example of this is the thought experiment surrounding Margo, an Alzheimer's patient who seems to live a perfectly pleasant life, but whose living will asks that no treatment be given. See President's Council on Bioethics, *Taking Care*, 82–88; Ronald Dworkin, *Life's Dominion: An Argument about Abortion, Euthanasia, and Individual Freedom* (New York: Vintage, 1994), 221–22; Rebecca Dresser, "Dworkin on Dementia: Elegant Theory, Questionable Policy," *Hastings Center Report* 25, no. 6 (November 12, 1995): 32–38.

15. Daniel Kahneman, *Thinking, Fast and Slow* (New York: Farrar, Straus and Giroux, 2013).

16. See the example of Maureen Peterson in Sharon R. Kaufman, *And a Time to Die: How American Hospitals Shape the End of Life* (Chicago: University of Chicago Press, 2006), 301.

17. Michael Banner, *The Ethics of Everyday Life* (New York: Oxford University Press, 2014), 107–34.

18. Barbara Coombs Lee, "Oregon's Experience with Aid in Dying: Findings from the Death with Dignity Laboratory," *Annals of the New York Academy of Sciences* 1330, no. 1 (November 2014): 94–100.

19. Of course other framings of suicide are possible in other cultures and in certain subcultures in our own societies, as shown in Lisa Stevenson, *Life Beside Itself* (Berkeley: University of California Press, 2014).

20. E.g., Bonnie Steinbock, "Physician-Assisted Death and Severe, Treatment-Resistant Depression," *Hastings Center Report* 47, no. 5 (September 1, 2017): 30–42.

21. For an insightful summary of such criticisms, see Verhey, *The Christian Art of Dying*, 59–67.

22. Anthony Fisher, *Catholic Bioethics for a New Millennium* (New York: Cambridge University Press, 2011), 289.

23. Alasdair MacIntyre, *Dependent Rational Animals: Why Human Beings Need the Virtues* (Chicago: Open Court, 1999).

24. President's Council on Bioethics, *Beyond Therapy: Biotechnology and the Pursuit of Happiness* (Washington, DC: President's Council on Bioethics, 2003), 287–90; Michael J. Sandel, *The Case against Perfection: Ethics in the Age of Genetic Engineering* (Cambridge, MA: Belknap Press, 2009).

25. For the origins of the ethics of care, see Carol Gilligan, *In a Different Voice: Psychological Theory and Women's Development* (Cambridge, MA: Harvard University Press, 2016).

26. Cicero, "De Senectute," in *On Old Age. On Friendship. On Divination*, Loeb Classical Library no. 154 (Cambridge, MA: Harvard University Press, 1923), II.4.

27. Mahmood, *Politics of Piety*, 129–30.

28. Phil. 2:6–8. Biblical citations are from the New American Bible, trans. Donald Senior and John J. Collins, eds., *The Catholic Study Bible*, 2nd ed. (New York: Oxford University Press, 2006).

29. For the connection between kenosis, suffering, and exaltation, see John Paul II, *Salvifici Doloris*, 1984, 22–23, https://w2.vatican.va/content/john-paul-ii/en/apost_letters/1984/documents/hf_jp-ii_apl_11021984_salvifici-doloris.html.

30. See Lucien Richard, "Toward a Theology of Aging," *Science et Esprit* 34, no. 3 (1982): 269–87. One finds a similar focus on the human passive agency of Christ, but from a different, Barthian, perspective, in Autumn Ridenour, "The Coming of Age: Curse or Calling? Toward a Christological Interpretation of Aging as Call in the Theology of Karl Barth and W. H. Vanstone," *Journal of the Society of Christian Ethics* 33, no. 2 (Fall/Winter 2013): 151–67.

31. Col. 1:24.

32. John Paul II, *Salvifici Doloris*, 31; Benedict XVI, *Spe Salvi* (Nairobi: Pauline Publications Africa, 2007), 40.

33. John Paul II, *Salvifici Doloris*, 27.

34. Ibid.

35. Janelle S. Taylor, "On Recognition, Caring, and Dementia," *Medical Anthropology Quarterly* 22, no. 4 (December 2, 2008): 313–35.

36. Michael Banner, "Scripts for Modern Dying: The Death before Death We Have Invented, the Death before Death We Fear and Some Take Too Literally, and the Death before Death Christians Believe In," *Studies in Christian Ethics* 29, no. 3 (August 1, 2016): 249–55. Banner's language here has to be taken carefully. The Catholic bioethical tradition, and many other Christian bioethics, do not accept that the cognitive decline associated with dementia can lead to the loss of personhood or truly even the loss of the self. In these traditions, the self and the person remain until bodily death, although in a diseased state. I take his language in a more metaphorical sense. Moreover, the death to the self that the person facing dementia accepts would have to be a conscious appropriation of their situation in light of the Cross.

37. Robert Desjarlais, *Subject to Death: Life and Loss in a Buddhist World* (Chicago: University of Chicago Press, 2016), 40.

38. Ibid., 41.

39. Martin Heidegger, *Being and Time*, trans. John MacQuarrie and Edward Robinson (New York: Harper and Row, 1962).

40. Hadot, *Philosophy as a Way of Life*.

41. Foucault, *The Hermeneutics of the Subject*, 466–73; Cicero, *Tusculan Disputations*, trans. J. E. King, Loeb Classical Library no. 141 (Cambridge, MA: Harvard University Press, 1927), III.14.

42. Paul Scherz, "Living Indefinitely and Living Fully: Laudato Si' and the Value of the Present in Christian, Stoic, and Transhumanist Temporalities," *Theological Studies* 79, no. 2 (June 2018): 356–75.

43. For a discussion of similarities and differences between Christian and Stoic attitudes toward death and the ways that these affected the *ars moriendi*, see Paul Scherz, "Grief, Death, and Longing in Stoic and Christian Ethics," *Journal of Religious Ethics* 45, no. 1 (February 2017): 7–28.

44. For broader discussions of this art of dying, see Verhey, *The Christian Art of Dying*; Christopher P. Vogt, *Patience, Compassion, Hope, and the Christian Art of Dying Well* (Lanham, MD: Rowman and Littlefield, 2004); Carlos M. N. Eire, *From Madrid to Purgatory: The Art and Craft of Dying in Sixteenth-Century Spain* (Cambridge: Cambridge University Press, 2002); Lydia Dugdale, ed., *Dying in the Twenty-First Century: Toward a New Ethical Framework for the Art of Dying Well* (Cambridge, MA: MIT Press, 2016).

45. Desiderius Erasmus, "Preparing for Death," in *Spiritualia and Pastoralia*, ed. John W. O'Malley, trans. John Grant, Collected Works of Erasmus vol. 70 (Toronto: University of Toronto Press, 1988), 389–450.

46. E.g., ibid., 398; Roberto Francesco Romolo Bellarmine, "The Art of Dying Well," in *Spiritual Writings*, trans. John Patrick Donnelly and Roland J. Teske,

Classics of Western Spirituality (New York: Paulist Press, 1989), 239. This insight has become the center of contemporary theological efforts to recover the art of dying, such as that in Vogt, *Patience, Compassion, Hope, and the Christian Art of Dying Well*, and Verhey, *The Christian Art of Dying*.

47. Erasmus, "Preparing for Death," 394; Bellarmine, "The Art of Dying Well," 243; Alphonsus Liguori, *Preparation for Death*, ed. Eugene Grimm (Brooklyn: Redemptorist Fathers, 1926), 44.

48. Erasmus, "Preparing for Death," 420; Liguori, *Preparation for Death*, 372–82.

49. Ps. 90:12.

PART II

Living Old Age Well

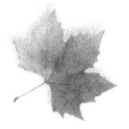

CHAPTER FOUR

Epiphanies, Small and Large

WILFRED M. McCLAY

The compulsive jokiness with which so many modern Americans deflect the subject of aging can get pretty tiresome. But it is perhaps not the worst way to handle the matter. It at least avoids the undignified excesses of self-pity and despair by making light of an admittedly unwelcome condition, even while implicitly confessing one's susceptibility to an all-too-human vanity. That was the approach taken by the great comedian Jack Benny, whose trademark shtick included the comic pretense that he was perpetually thirty-nine. There was irony built into the joke, a self-mockery that was at least honest enough to acknowledge itself. That way, we could identify with it too. Laughing at Jack Benny, we were also laughing at ourselves; he was so much like us, merely offering up a silly and exaggerated version of what so many of us are tempted to do.

But even great comedy has its limits. A jokey evasion is still an evasion, one that not only tries to hide a great deal of anxiety, but also distracts us from seeking the deeper meanings in our experience. A joke may be a very civilized way of coping, but it is not an answer to much of anything, and it may even be a veiled way of confessing to the dread that there are no answers to be had. "I'm not afraid of death," said Woody Allen, "I just don't want to be there when it happens." A very funny line, but what makes it so funny is the way that it confirms the overwhelming force of the very fear it claims to deny.

Yet there is a grain of wisdom to be found in the ironic reversal that these jokes perform. It points back to a deep and persistent insight of our civilization: the teaching that the structure of human growth is itself paradoxical, a startling play of reversals in which opposites trade places and the loss of something ordinary becomes the path to the acquisition of something higher and rarer. St. Paul described a God whose power was "made perfect in weakness," perhaps the quintessential formulation of the paradox; but the insight is not exclusive to Christianity. In writers from Homer to Sophocles to Milton, blindness leads to the profounder form of vision. Loss is gain, diminution is increase, woundedness produces strength, disability opens the door to extraordinary ability, wisdom is shown as foolishness and foolishness as wisdom. Holding too tightly to a proximate good can block our way to the appropriation of something far better.

There are a multitude of lessons in this for an age in which the steady advance of the sovereign human will, embodied in the mastery of nature by medical science, seems to be yielding a harvest of surprising barrenness: anxiety, loneliness, purposelessness, anomie. One of the lessons is that we need, contra Woody Allen, to be there for the whole journey. Disembodiment and distraction during the latter parts will not do the job. There are certain subtle and almost inexpressible little epiphanies that come to us with the advance of age, but you have to be paying attention if you are to catch them. Let me describe one such epiphany by way of illustration. I won't try to give it a name, since it is easier to describe than to formulate or define.

So then, let me create a scene for your mind's eye. Imagine yourself as a young man, perhaps in late adolescence or early adulthood. In the course of events—perhaps sitting in the seat beside you on an airplane flight—you meet a little old lady. At least that is how you unreflectively categorize her, both when you meet her and when you describe her later to your friends: a little old lady. Since you are (obviously) a bit callow, it doesn't even cross your mind to think that characterization might be a bit slighting or callous. After all, you mean no harm. But even if your perception of her is positive, it is also casually reductive, a stereotype without any shade of complexity or shadow of turning. Someone else might have noticed that she is a lively conversationalist and is impeccably dressed and coiffed, with perfectly manicured nails, but none of that registers with you. Instead, you mainly see her as someone standing at a certain remove from you, as a second-grader sees his teacher, across a continental divide of age, having long ago arrived at that great gray stage of human life in which the imperatives of youth, the only imperatives you really understand, are as distant from hers as those of someone in the Middle Ages.

Needless to say, this little scenario is all going to look quite different to the woman. She undoubtedly doesn't think of herself as a Little Old Lady, if for no other reason than that no one wants to be reduced to a stereotype. But there are likely many other reasons. Perhaps she doesn't like to be reminded of her age, doesn't feel that she is all that "old," or, for that matter, isn't little and doesn't feel much like a lady at the moment. Or she is too busy thinking about other things and would find the label attached to her by an ignorant boy uninteresting. Or amusing. Or impertinent, an example of the oafish imperialism of youth in our culture. There are plenty of other reasons for her to find it an inaccurate or annoying label. But the one-dimensional reductionism of it is the heart of the matter.

Now instead imagine being a male contemporary of that same woman, someone she had known years before, perhaps in another place, but had only rarely or never seen in the intervening years. In fact, let's say that you two were college friends, and you bump into one another at a reunion event. You sit down to have a cup of coffee and talk. And you proceed not only to talk, running through the usual updates of marriage, children, careers, relocations, medical problems, etc., but to look carefully at one another as you do. What are you looking for? What do you see? What impressions flow into your mind in silent counterpoint to the words coming out of your mouth?

Of course you look for and see many things. But first of all, you search for the face of the person you used to know as it appears in the face of the person who now sits across from you. And once you recognize it, once that face of the younger person emerges in a way visible to you, you cannot unsee it; you cannot see her today in any other way, without also incorporating that younger person, without that almost ghostly presence inhering in the sight. You come into possession of a kind of dual vision. You look in her face and see not only the face that she has now, but also the face she had then, even if it only peeks out here and there in fleeting moments or shows itself in certain tics and mannerisms that have endured. You experience her as a life in motion.

You might have a variety of reactions to the changes that have occurred over the years—the human body being what it is, the changes will generally look like wear and tear, at best—but what can't be helped is that, in some sense, both people are alive to you at that moment. The person you used to know is still alive somewhere in there. You can detect that spark and hear that distant melody. You can see what the young man is incapable of seeing: that this is no mere little old lady. In the house of her soul are many mansions; as the governess tells the young lovers in *The King and I*, she "knows how it feels to have wings on your heels, and to fly down the street in a trance." Not that she is ever likely to do that again. But in some sense, she never ceased to be what she was, in the process of becoming what she is now.

That is the epiphany, then. It is the understanding, not only as an abstract idea but as a living reality, that a human person is a historical being in whom the past remains immanent in the present, a human being whom the passage of time enhances as much as it diminishes. We rarely are presented with exactly the right circumstances to gain this insight, although occasions such as reunions are perfect places for them to occur; and of course you can get an intimation of it from family photos and videos in which you glimpse what your now-wizened grandparents looked like when they were twenty-somethings and newly married.

But once one has gained the insight, one can begin to generalize from it. It is not just this one person who can be seen and understood doubly. We can train the insight onto the faces of others, even others we do not know. Even little old men on airplanes. It becomes a kind of solitary parlor game. We can look at their faces and extrapolate what they might have looked like if we had known them when they were young. Or we can look at the faces of the young and imagine them as they might appear someday when they have grown old.

One of the great poems about aging, William Butler Yeats's "Among School Children," describes something very similar to this and features a similar epiphany. The author is visiting a classroom full of industrious little children and finds himself being stared at by them as "a sixty-year-old smiling public man"—a stereotypical little old man, as it were. But like the young man on the airplane, those little kids have no idea of how much wild subjectivity is going on beneath that bland exterior. His mind is racing. He is thinking passionate thoughts about a woman he loves, how they bonded over her recounting of a childhood wound that she had received—and then he looks at the children in the class and wonders "if she stood so at that age" and realizes, with a start, that any one of these girls might be having experiences similar to hers and might eventually grow up to be like her. "And thereupon," he exclaims, "my heart is driven wild: / She stands before me as a living child."

But he does not stop there. He then reflects on his beloved's once-beautiful but now much-diminished face, fifty or more years older than that of these schoolgirls, "hollow of cheek as though it drank the wind / And took a mess of shadows for its meat"—a face that has become marked, that is, with the wear and tear of a sad and difficult life. Such a dismaying thought then leads him to wonder whether it is worth it all, even to be born. After all, what mother would consent even to give birth to a child in the first place, were she to know in advance that her once-perfect child would end up looking like this? Or like him, for that matter, a mere "scarecrow" of a man at sixty years?

He was posing one of the core questions about aging. How can the mounting debilities of old age—the loss of beauty, mobility, strength, mental acuity, sexual charm, and so many other losses—be understood as anything more than the terrible sadness and pity that attaches to all human flesh once it passes a certain marker (say, thirty-nine)? And, like all questions of aging, it quickly becomes a question about the value of life itself. Why bring new life into the world at all, why endure and strive and struggle, if that new life is destined for failure and disappointment in maturity, and then on, cut by cut, to an ignominious end, sans teeth, sans eyes, sans taste, sans everything?

He does not provide an answer. Yet he provides the beginnings of one in the form of a question posed as the poem concludes: "O chestnut tree, great rooted blossomer, / Are you the leaf, the blossom or the bole?"

I think the question answers itself. The chestnut tree is all three of these things, and many others besides. Its organic life is a continuous succession of stages, and while one or another stage may be the most prized by us—say, the blossom stage—none exists apart from the others. The human person, in his or her completeness, is not one stage or another, but all of them together, time past and time present containing time future.

Hence the dilemma we face when we have to choose a photograph to accompany an obituary, our usual way of trying to sum up a life. Do we choose the picture of the blossoming young graduate, the newly commissioned officer, the bride or the groom—a picture of someone full of promise, but whom no one reading the paper will recognize? Or do we choose the robust thirty-nine-year-old, the mature fifty-year-old, or the seventy-year-old, the little old man or woman whose picture a few in the community will recognize when they see it? Which best represents the person in his or her wholeness?

I faced this dilemma myself a number of years ago when I had to provide the newspapers with an obituary photograph of my recently deceased mother. In the end, I was prevailed upon by family members to provide a youthful photo, and they probably were right to insist upon that. An obituary is not the moment to challenge social conventions. But if I could have had my druthers, I would have chosen a photo from her old age. To explain why will, I think, be a useful way to go more deeply into the question that hovers over the evening of life: How can the latter stages of life be a time of crucial illumination in which loss becomes gain and disability becomes strength? The answer to this question is precisely the insight we so badly need to regain as we think about the status of aging in our increasingly barren culture of material mastery. So I hope the reader will indulge my trying to make the point by way of some extended personal reminiscences.

Let me begin by relating something my mother said to me once in a conversation we had early in my days as a graduate student in history at Johns Hopkins. I mentioned to her that I'd just read a biography of H. L. Mencken, the irreverent and merciless editor and critic known as the "sage of Baltimore." I had never known that Mencken had suffered a stroke while still in his prime and spent his last years unable to write or read and only barely able to speak. This must have been, for him, like being a shark without teeth. I remarked on the fact that this particular biographer had almost nothing to say about that part of Mencken's life—how Mencken adapted, if he did, to his disability and, more generally, how it affected him. Did it do anything to change his outlook, cause him to moderate his tone, rethink his slashing critical style? That wasn't addressed at all. It was an astonishing omission, to my mind. It really was as if, for all practical purposes, Mencken's life was deemed to be over when he had the stroke.

My mother responded, somewhat out of the blue, that she wanted me to know that if *she* ever found herself in a condition similar to that of Mencken, she hoped that I would do nothing to prolong her life, because a life lived that way would not be worth living. It was a slightly chilling statement, particularly coming out of the blue and matter-of-fact in that way, but she absolutely meant it. I could tell she did. I don't mean that she was a social Darwinist, thought the weak and infirm should be allowed to perish, or anything like that. She was always generous and warmhearted with people, particularly those in her inner circle—family and friends of family.

But she was a mathematician who believed in being unflinchingly honest about things that other people are willing to blur, and her statement, which she made with a mathematician's crisp rationality, was completely consistent with her view of life. She was saying that, absent a certain "quality of life," there was no point in living. There was certainly no reason that we, the healthy, should go to great lengths to support and extend the lives of those who are severely impaired. And to be fair, I think her view at that time was only a more honest expression of sentiments that are held by many, maybe even most, modern Americans, though rarely expressed with the honesty and directness she showed that day. We assume that we know what it is that we want and need in life and that we must be the masters of our own faculties to achieve it.

But it was only a couple of years later that my mother herself suffered a massive stroke that nearly killed her, and, once she emerged from a month-long coma, left her with an enormous loss of cognitive function and, in particular, an inability to speak, write, or read. I remember a particular moment, as she was emerging from her coma, when the enormity of what had happened seemed suddenly to bear down on her. She was hit with a realization of the huge gulf that now separated her, forever, from the person that she had been—the highly verbal, articulate, and independent-minded mathematician, reader, teacher, mother, puzzle-solver, bridge-player, and vivacious conversationalist. All that she was most proud of in herself was gone. That self was now dead. And at that moment she cried, with the deepest, most grief-laden, most soul-wrenching sobs and moans I've ever heard in my life. I can still hear them in my mind, and I can never forget that moment.

But that wasn't the end of the story. After a period of rehabilitation, she was able to return home. Eventually she was even able to live on her own, with significant assistance for meal preparation and housecleaning. She was able to live a reasonably satisfying life in the house she loved. True, many things were missing, and it was often lonely. Perhaps the greatest disappointment was the loss of the company of so many of her friends, who found it so hard to be around her in her changed condition and just never visited. Her whole world had contracted to a handful of people, most of them immediate family members, chiefly my sister, my wife, my children, and me.

Someone writing her biography might have concluded, like Mencken's biographer, that there was nothing to say about those years and that her life was effectively over. Actually, something closer to the opposite was true. There was an inner development going on in her during those years that was absolutely remarkable to behold. She became a far deeper, warmer, more affectionate, more grateful, and more generous person than I had ever known her to be. It is always a mystery why some people respond to adversity by closing themselves off, while others respond by opening their hearts; she did the latter. In some respects, we became closer than we had ever been. She actually had lost very little of her intellectual capacity, only the ability to express her thoughts readily, and by working together we found a hundred different ways of working around the barriers. She had a very small working vocabulary and could almost never string words together into sentences, but no human being who has walked the planet has ever done more with a few words or been able to express more intricate shades of meaning simply by intoning the same words differently. She even had the ability to make light of her own verbal habits, such as the use of an impatient "OK!" that she used to say, in effect, that's enough, let's move on to another subject. And I think it pleased her to no end that we all picked up her mannerisms and used them all the time. Another person might have perceived that as an insult, but she delighted in it.

And, perhaps the most surprising thing of all, she proved to be a fantastic grandmother to my two children, whom she loved without reservation and who loved her the same way in return. That meant so much to her, precisely because she knew that you can't force kids to be loving toward their grandparents. She knew they weren't faking it and knew they didn't treat her well merely because they felt sorry for her. Being almost completely helpless and dependent, she was not able to bribe their affections with illicit candy and other such allurements the way grandmothers have done since time immemorial. She had no weapon other than herself. Thankfully, my children always saw past her disability, recognized her awesome depth of character, and admired her without reservation. What they couldn't possibly know was how much they did to help make life worth living for her. If she ever doubted her capacity to be a first-rate grandmother, and I know that she did at times, the kids dissipated that doubt in a jiffy, just by the easy and unfeigned everyday way they treated her.

She came to live with me and my family in Tennessee during her last years, when a series of subsequent strokes had made it impossible for her to live on her own and we knew that we couldn't even consider putting her in a nursing home. She had to be with her own. It wasn't always easy, of course, and while I don't want to dwell on the details of that, I don't want to pretend that it wasn't a strain. But there are so many memories of those years that we treasure—above all, the day-in and day-out experience of my mother's great and unbowed spirit, which inspired and awed us all. She made me think often of a different verse by Yeats, from "Sailing to Byzantium":

> An aged man is but a paltry thing
> A tattered coat upon a stick
> Unless soul clap its hands, and sing
> And louder sing for every tatter in its mortal dress.

Well, my mother did clap and sing, and she did it every single day, whether her body wanted to cooperate or not. And although she had every reason to be bitter, she wasn't. Her song was joyful, gracious, grateful, and infectious. She learned to take infinite pleasure in the simplest of things — the antics of our dogs, the taste of good food, the sound of the piano, the busy birds at the feeder, the turning of the leaves, the whisper of the wind in the trees — and to see these things as the immense gifts that they are. Being around her, seeing the joy she took in these things, you couldn't help but share those feelings and feel lifted out of ordinary concerns and worries into something much closer to the whole truth about our miraculous world. It took a long time to adjust to the silence in the house when she was gone.

I could say much more, but the lesson is this: that when we talk about "the quality of life," we need to think more carefully about what we mean. By most people's standards, the last twenty years of my mother's life were like the last years of Mencken's — dark, sad years spent waiting for the curtain to fall on a drama that was essentially over. But those of us who were privileged to know her in those years know better. Her stroke was not only an end, but also a beginning. And that is true of every one of life's junctures, no matter how painful or frightening or sad it may seem when we go through it.

I will always remember my mother in every phase of her life with fondness and joy, including even the phase of my own early life, of which I have the faintest memories, when she loomed as large and powerful as a titan. But I will especially treasure these last years, watching her tread a very hard and weary path with a grace and joy that I could never hope to equal. Her power was being made perfect in her weakness. When I think of the term "quality of life," that is what I will remember. For her, the evening of the body became a morning of the spirit.

What does one woman's story prove? Anecdotes are not data, as they say; but data are not life. There are numerous lessons to be drawn from this story, but surely at the very top of the list would be this one: that our drive for mastery of the terms of our existence, as heroic and noble as its achievements have been, may also be the enemy of our souls. Aging is not a problem to be solved but a meaning to be lived out. I don't think my mother's case was unique or needs to be. And I don't think it requires a cultural revolution for things to change. But we do need to open ourselves to many more epiphanies, small and large.

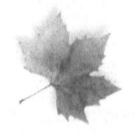

CHAPTER FIVE

The Contraction of Time and Existential Awakening
A Phenomenology of Authentic Aging

KEVIN AHO

An oft-cited study by palliative care nurse Bronnie Ware examined the biggest regrets that people have on their deathbeds, revealing some interesting things about the ways in which we prioritize our lives when we are young and healthy. Regrets include these: "I wish I didn't work so hard," "I wish I had the courage to express my feelings," "I wish I had stayed in touch with friends," and "I wish that I let myself be happier." But, according to this study, the most profound disappointment experienced as we move toward death involves the issue of authenticity, of *being true* to oneself. In confronting the end of their lives, participants made this regret clear: "I wish I'd had the courage to live a life true to myself [and] not the life others expected of me."[1] Although the study seems to suggest that by the time one is physically incapacitated or on their deathbed it is too late for authenticity, I want to offer an alternative account. Drawing on a phenomenological interpretation of time and insights from social psychology and existential philosophy, my aim is to show how the experience of aging and decline, while certainly accompanied by the pains of physical diminishment, personal loss, and various forms of regret, can also awaken us to the possibility for what can be called "authentic aging" by freeing us from trivial concerns, enabling deeper and more profound forms of interpersonal communication, and prompting an awareness of the fragility and preciousness of the present moment. By regarding the future as a horizon of existential possibilities and interpreting aging as the inevitable narrowing and tightening of this horizon, I hope to show how the experience of temporal contraction, if received properly, can push away banal distractions and light up what genuinely matters in our lives.

Ageism and Death Anxiety

A recent article in the *New Yorker* documents the ubiquitous "ageism" running rampant in Silicon Valley, the epicenter of the new information economy. The author references Mark Zuckerberg, who created Facebook at the age of nineteen and claims that "young people are just smarter." And also Sun Microsystem's co-founder Vinod Khosla, who suggests that "people over forty-five basically die in terms of new ideas."[2] What has become clear with the burgeoning economic and political power of "the Valley" is that ageism, manifesting in tandem with our current obsessions with youth and beauty, is not only here to stay; it is getting worse. Understood as a negative judgment toward the processes of aging and of older adults in general, the current expression of ageism is being conveyed culturally through a wide range of media platforms, including movies and television, social media, self-help books, magazines, and advertising. The negative stereotype generally suggests that the elderly are, among other things, socially and technologically incompetent, have diminished cognitive functioning, are no longer physically desirable or sexually active, and are lonely and depressed. And it is thought that when these stereotypes are internalized, the result is decreased self-esteem, self-efficacy, and overall life satisfaction.[3]

But what distinguishes ageism from other "isms"—such as sexism or racism—is that it is directed not toward an amorphous "other" with a different gender, sexual orientation, or skin tone, but toward our own future self. Understood this way, ageism looks like a kind of self-hatred of who we will one day become. This means that the elderly today probably participated in the same negative stereotyping that they are now being subjected to. This hostility toward our future selves raises interesting questions for the prospect of authenticity. If authenticity, as the Greek word *authentikos* suggests, has something to do with being "genuine" or "true" to one's self, and the self is not just who we are today but who we *will be*, ageism looks like a form of dishonesty or self-denial. The existentialist tradition is especially helpful here because it generally frames authenticity in terms of a steadfast willingness to be open to and accepting of one's own temporal constitution. In this view, inauthenticity involves an unwillingness to accept our future selves because of what that self represents: physical decay, illness, cognitive decline, public humiliations, and, ultimately, death. To the extent that we are shaped by ageist stereotypes, the process of growing older and the elderly themselves represent something that is profoundly unsettling—a threat to our very being. The work of Ernest Becker and the Terror Management Theory (TMT) he inspired provides insight into this pervasive phenomenon of self-denial.[4]

Following in the existentialist tradition, Becker and TMT suggest that the core burden of our condition derives from the distinctly human capacity for self-awareness, that we are conscious of our existence and driven to live but at the same time understand that our existence is finite and constantly threatened by the possibility of death. The terror that emerges from this tension—the desire to live clashing with the reality of death—is controlled and managed through symbolic practices and cultural institutions that we are habituated into and that enable us to repress and deny our own existential reality. This denial is expressed in any number of ways—through belief in God and the immortality of the soul, for example, through having children, accumulating wealth, clinging to occupational titles or social roles, or leaving a legacy. Each of these symbolic mechanisms, in their own way, serves as an immortality project, sheltering us from the terror of death by creating the illusion of stability and permanence. Ageism, manifesting in our cultural obsession with youth and negative views of the elderly, is another example.

TMT has explored different ways in which the death anxiety aroused by aging and the elderly is pushed back into the unconscious.[5] The most obvious strategy is to simply avoid them. By physically staying away from places where the elderly congregate, such as senior centers, golf courses, doctors' offices, and bingo parlors, we can protect ourselves from the reminder of death. Similarly, we can try to keep the elderly out of the workforce or place our aging relatives in nursing homes or assisted living communities to reduce our exposure to old age and death. Jeff Greenberg and his colleagues go on to point out how patterns of physical distancing can often lead to more insidious forms of psychological distancing whereby we dehumanize the elderly, failing to acknowledge them as persons by identifying them with demeaning terms such as "geezer," "old timer," or "blue hair."[6] This allows one to view the elderly as somehow different from oneself, as less than human. And this, in turn, can increase one's self-esteem by strengthening the ageist worldview, namely, that we are not like the elderly, and the devastations of aging belong to the elderly, not to oneself. Following the existentialist conception of authenticity, I want to suggest that these defense mechanisms involve a form of self-denial that can be overcome only by becoming aware of our own mortality, which involves accepting the extent to which our existence is constituted by time. Accepting and "being true" to our temporal constitution not only diminishes the threat of death; it also opens up productive ways to integrate the unique forms of wisdom and meaning that aging can bring to our everyday lives.

Aging as Temporal Contraction

By articulating the inescapable finitude of the human condition, notable existentialist thinkers such as Martin Heidegger provide a unique perspective from which to access the experience of aging. Although he never discusses the issue of aging in his work and rarely even mentions the fact that human existence (or *Dasein*) is embodied, Heidegger's thought is significant in forwarding the idea that Dasein should not be viewed as an objectively present substance or thing.[7] It is, rather, a self-interpreting activity or event that is structured by time. In this view, the temporal aspects of past and future are not datable "now-points" that can be located on a clock or calendar. They are, rather, conditions or structures that constitute our being (or identity), that is, the interpretation or understanding that we have of ourselves. This means that time is not something external to us that can be measured or saved. This ordinary conception of clock time is derived from and parasitic on a more primordial conception, that of existential or lived time. Existential time is not *something we have*; it is *who we are*. "Time is Dasein," as Heidegger says, "[and] Dasein is time."[8] From the perspective of aging, then, time has little to do with one's chronological age or even the time of changing biological processes, menopause, erectile dysfunction, or cognitive decline. It is a reference, rather, to a future that is narrowing or contracting, forcing out possibilities that are no longer livable. This conception of temporal contraction is perhaps best grasped with Heidegger's interpretation of human existence as "thrown projection" (*geworfen Entwurf*). Here, to be human is to be "thrown" into a contingent past, into a shared sociohistorical situation that we cannot get behind, and it is against the background of this situation that a future is opened up, revealing a horizon of possibilities that we can "project" for ourselves. And it is through these historically mediated projects that we come to understand and make sense of who we are. When Heidegger says we are "thrown into the kind of being which we call projecting," he is describing how our existence or self-interpretation is always "running ahead" of itself, pressing forward into future possibilities but always against the constraints and limitations of our past.[9] Thus, in Heidegger's words, "running ahead to the past is Dasein's possibility of Being; [it] *is time itself*."[10]

When we are young and healthy, the horizon of future projects is expansive, revealing a broad range of possibilities that we can seamlessly press into. Whether it is choosing to embark on a new career, changing relationship status, learning a new sport, or moving to a different part of the country, the future promises a vast array of options through which we can fashion and refashion our self-interpretations. At this stage in life, our orientation is largely acquisitive, shaped by a desire for novelty, as we reach out for new information, adventures, and material possessions. In *Being and Time*, Heidegger refers to this attitude in terms of "curiosity" (*Neugier*), whereby we are carried away by the latest distractions and fads of the day, "seek[ing] novelty only in order to leap from it anew to another novelty."[11] This acquisitive attitude generally assumes that time is expansive and unlimited. But as we age, the expansiveness of our future begins to contract, gradually closing off possibilities that are no longer viable for us. This experience of contraction can be terrifying, triggering an awareness of our temporal constitution and often resulting in the so-called "midlife crisis."

The experience of such a crisis is, of course, a relatively recent phenomenon, due in large part to a radical change in the average span of life in the West. In the late nineteenth century, the life expectancy was about forty years, and one's adult life was devoted largely to work, marriage, and raising children. By the time the last child left the house, the parents were already close to death if not dead already. Today, the life expectancy for Americans is near eighty, providing ample time to reflect on one's contracting future. These kinds of reflections can result in predictable midlife experiences and behaviors, from a newfound obsession with nutrition, exercise, sex, and losing weight in an effort to look and feel younger and more vital to the depressing feeling of being trapped, whether it is in the same job for another twenty years before retirement or in a marriage that has been stripped of the essential meanings associated with child rearing. As one woman writes:

> It's unbelievable when I think of it now. I never really saw past about age forty-two, where I am now. I mean I never thought about what happens to the rest of life. Pretty much the whole adult life was supposed to be around your husband and raising children. Dammit, what a betrayal! Nobody ever tells you that there [are] many years of life after children are raised. Now what?[12]

Although forty-two is hardly old, the crisis of meaning the woman is describing and the myriad age-denying behaviors that begin to manifest at midlife may actually be a response to a dormant anxiety that erupts when we confront our own finitude. From the perspective of existentialist thought, these kinds of emotional crises are unique insofar as they have the power to disclose fundamental truths of the human condition. The woman's anxiety, in the existentialist account, is directed not necessarily at her now childless life but at her own structural impermanence, at *the nothing* at the core of her existence. The crisis reveals that any sense of stability and constancy regarding the identity she has established over many years of mothering was an illusion. When her children left home, her world collapsed and the meaning and coherence of her identity were stripped away. She was exposed to her own contingency, to the fact that there is nothing enduring or lasting about her being. This is why Heidegger says, "[*Human existence*] *itself is that in the face of which anxiety is anxious.*"[13]

Although the collapse of meaning can be terrifying, the existentialists suggest that it also presents an opportunity by shaking us out of the false security of everyday life. By reminding us of our fundamental contingency and finitude, the crisis can awaken us to our own nothingness, to a future that is no longer expanding, no longer holding open a wide array of possibilities. Authenticity, in this view, involves facing and owning up to the crisis and integrating it into our lives rather than fleeing back into our secure routines. Such acceptance opens up a space for personal and spiritual growth by forcing us to confront the fact that our time is limited and cannot be taken for granted. When our future is genuinely grasped as precarious and contracting rather than endlessly open and expanding, it can shift our orientation and illuminate the ultimate questions: "Who am I?" and "What is the purpose of my life?" Answering these transformative questions makes it possible for us to face ourselves, to rearrange and adjust our choices and priorities in ways that can deepen and enhance experiences of well-being and interpersonal connection. Evidence of this kind of growth can often be found in the social networks and communicative practices of the elderly.

Relational Depth and Vulnerability

Social psychologists working in an area called Socioemotional Selectivity Theory (SST) have suggested that, as the future contracts during the aging process, we often become more selective in our social commitments and projects, investing in interpersonal relationships and forms of communication that are more intimate and emotionally rich.[14] When one's own time is grasped as contracting rather than expanding, there is a tendency to withdraw from the vast social networks of our youth and interactions based largely on acquisitive novelty, gossip, and distraction. Older adults usually have smaller and more close-knit social networks. The assumption of SST is that in recognizing their own limited time, they would rather avoid superficial encounters with strangers, acquaintances, or colleagues, preferring the deep and emotionally satisfying connections of family and close friends. And through this kind of selectivity of social partners, they are often able to maintain more positive emotions.[15]

The existentialist conception of authenticity deepens this insight by focusing our awareness on the fundamental vulnerability at the core of the human condition. In terms of communicative practices, this awareness generally results in avoiding the petty gossip and ego-driven quarrels that can dominate so much of our everyday discourse. With a contracting future, these trivial issues are seen as irrelevant, as "wastes of time," and are replaced with forms of communication that honestly engage the limitations and frailties of being human. Oregon Senator Richard Neuberger describes this experience of discursive transformation in confronting and accepting his own finitude in the wake of a cancer diagnosis:

> A change came over me which I believe is irreversible. . . . My wife and I have not had a quarrel since my illness was diagnosed. I used to scold her for squeezing the toothpaste from the top instead of the bottom, about not catering sufficiently to my fussy appetite, about making up guest lists without consulting, about spending too much on clothes. Now I am either unaware of such matters or they seem irrelevant.[16]

In owning up to his contracting future, Senator Neuberger became more focused on the poignancy of the present moment. No longer preoccupied with past slights or future ambitions, he acknowledged that time with his wife was finite, and he was more vulnerable and empathic, concerned with cultivating emotional intimacy and connection with her rather than quarreling about toothpaste. The upshot is that when we accept our finitude, we become more vulnerable and honest with ourselves and surround ourselves with others who are similarly vulnerable and honest. Chatting about politics, sports, relationship drama, social status, or money is often viewed as trivial and irrelevant, and the focus of conversation shifts to issues of deep meaning, opening ourselves up to our fears and insecurities and the existential concerns that matter deeply to us. Accessing this dimension of communicative depth often emerges in tandem with a transformation of the tempo or velocity of life as we age, a slowing down that makes it possible to be present and attend to the vulnerability of the other person.

Slowness and Presence

One of the more familiar ways in which we shield ourselves from death anxiety is through busyness. By remaining in constant motion and consumed by the ubiquitous distractions of technology, travel, work, shopping, and social events, we simply don't have the time to confront our finitude. In his later writings, Heidegger identifies this kind of evasion as one of the signature features of modern life, referring to it in terms of "acceleration" (*Schnelligkeit*), a kind of restlessness in which we are "not-able-to-bear the stillness" of our own lives. As in his account of "curiosity" in *Being and Time*, he describes acceleration as a kind of "mania for what is surprising, for what immediately sweeps [us] away and impresses [us] again and again and in different ways."[17] For Heidegger, this is a "fallen" (*verfallen*) or inauthentic mode of time, in which we are immersed in the harried pace of everyday life and oblivious to our own temporal constitution. In inauthentic time we crave newness and distraction and are scattered and dispersed in the curiosities of the moment. The result, in Heidegger's words, is that we are *"never-dwelling-anywhere."*[18] But aging provides an opportunity to dwell by breaking out of this accelerated cycle.

The physical decline and loss of strength and cognitive dexterity that accompany the aging process make it increasingly difficult to be pulled apart by everyday novelties and distractions. The elderly often cannot keep up with the speed of modern life, and this invariably shrinks the space of their daily concerns and opens up a void of stillness that can be terrifying. But if we can accept and integrate the slowness of aging into our lives rather than deny it, our own organic diminution has the power to open us to the dwelling place of the present moment so that we can attend to the things that are right in front of us. Heidegger refers to this kind of mindful attentiveness in terms of being in "the nearness" (*die Nähe*).[19] Rather than filling the stillness with more busyness, authentic aging involves, what Heidegger calls an "expectant decisiveness to be patient . . . [and] *the courage to go slowly.*"[20] Slowness, in this sense, can awaken us to the moment-to-moment experiences that we all too often take for granted when we are speeding through our lives. And this awakening illuminates the precariousness of both our existence and of the present moment. In patiently attending to what is near, the most ordinary and mundane encounters—a conversation with a friend, a cup of coffee in the morning, the cat purring on the couch, or flowers blooming in the spring—we can experience these things with "wonder" (*Erstaunen*), where the ordinary is experienced as extraordinary. "Wonder," as Heidegger puts it, "sets us before the usual itself [but] precisely as what is the most unusual."[21] Understood this way, slowing down and attending to what is near is a signal not of decay and diminishment, but of rebirth. It allows us to see the world with eyes that are fresh and new, with the eyes of a beginner. This explains why Martin Buber, in describing his own experience of aging, says that "to be old is a glorious thing when one has not unlearned what it means *to begin*. This old man had perhaps first learned it thoroughly in old age."[22]

Slowing down and seeing the world through beginners' eyes allows us to appreciate the transiency and impermanence of all things, including ourselves. This awareness can shake us out of inauthentic time, out of the comforting illusion that the future is far off in the distance and that life can be indefinitely postponed and deferred until "later." Frances, a nursing home resident, describes the experience of personal transformation that emerges when he accepts the slowing down and stillness that come with physical decline:

> Lack of physical strength keeps me inactive and often silent. They call me senile, but senility is just a convenient peg on which to hang non-conformity. A new set of faculties seems to be coming into operation. More than at any other time of my life I seem to be aware of the beauties of our spinning planet and the sky above. Old age is sharpening my Awareness.[23]

By slowing down and becoming aware of the fragility and impermanence of things, Frances is able to grasp the poignant beauty of life. In Heidegger's words, he has come to recognize the mysterious and extraordinary fact that "there is something rather than nothing, that there are beings and we ourselves are in their midst."[24] The intensifying and heightening of experience that comes from living slowly and being present not only disrupts the evasive habits of inauthentic time; it can also serve a liberating function as we age, freeing us from the ego-driven fears, ambitions, and preoccupations that torment us when we are young.

Freedom and Letting Go

Acknowledging that the future is contracting and that one's time is limited can help put life's priorities in perspective. Things that used to consume us when we were younger—our obsessions with income, our jobs, the kinds of cars we drive, or our physical appearance—no longer have the same power over us. Social psychologists have described this as an "accommodative shift," whereby the elderly begin to let go of the acquisitive goals and ambitions of their youth and adopt ones that are more compatible with the limited and restricted capacities of their later years.[25] But existentialist thought offers deeper insight into this capacity for letting go and why we are so preoccupied with these ego-driven projects in the first place. When Heidegger proclaims that "the 'essence' of Dasein lies in its existence," he is making it clear that human existence should not be viewed in terms of the objective presence of a physical substance or thing.[26] What is distinctive about Dasein is the fact that our being is an *issue* for us and that we are concerned about and care for our being. And this concern is expressed in the ongoing decisions we make as our lives unfold. Human existence, in this view, is a continuous process of self-making or self-fashioning whereby we are endlessly choosing ourselves, interpreting and giving meaning to the question of who we are. The fact that I am self-making in this way not only illuminates the future or forward-directedness of my existence; it also reveals that I am not a secure or self-subsisting thing but a *being possible*.

Because our existence is invariably "running ahead" into the possibilities we project for ourselves, it is structurally incomplete or "unfinished." As long as we exist, we are a "potentiality," a "no-thing." This is why Heidegger says, "[Dasein] must always, as such a potentiality, *not yet be* something."[27] This means that any identity or self-interpretation we happen to choose or create for ourselves is structurally vulnerable; our being is contingent and finite; it is a kind of nullity. As the horizon of possibilities contracts with age, we are bound to confront this vulnerability, recognizing that the sense of stability and permanence that our self-fashioning projects provide for us is an illusion. When we are inauthentic, we flee from this vulnerability and stubbornly cling to the public identities we have created for ourselves, deceiving ourselves into thinking that we are enduring and "real." But clinging in this way makes the aging process especially problematic because—in the wake of physical decline, illness, retirement, or the loss of loved ones—we are often unable to embody or perform our identities in the same way. As we saw earlier, the mother who devoted her life to child rearing can no longer interpret herself in the same way once the children become adults and leave home. So in order to be authentic or true to herself, she can no longer cling to this identity; she has to be willing to let it go. Heidegger will refer to this aspect of authenticity in terms of "resoluteness" (*Entschlossenheit*), where this is understood as a steadfast readiness to die, that is, to give up on identities that are no longer livable. *Entschlossenheit* conveys the literal sense of "being unlocked" or "open" to the nothingness at the core of the human condition, and this suggests a willingness to be free and flexible with our self-interpretations. Thus, in Heidegger's words, authentic Dasein "cannot become rigid as regards the situation, but must understand that resolution . . . must be held open and free for the current factical possibility."[28]

Understood this way, aging can be interpreted and experienced as a kind of liberation from the illusion of our own permanence and self-subsistence. Our youthful and middle-aged obsessions with money, productivity, social status, and physical appearance that serve to sustain this illusion become increasingly irrelevant as we move into old age. When confronted with our own nullity, we come to recognize that there was no enduring and stable self to begin with and that we have, at bottom, a finite existence, a vulnerable and tenuous process of self-creation. Following Heidegger's lead, existential psychiatrist Irvin Yalom found that when his patients accepted this truth they often felt released from their ego-driven fears of failure and rejection.[29] Many came to recognize that the primary source of their suffering emerged as a result of fleeing from their own finitude rather than accepting it. By stubbornly clinging to their identities and denying the fundamental transiency and impermanence of things, his patients led more fearful and constricted lives. When they were capable of letting go of this tendency, their lives opened up and their experiences were colored with a renewed sense of urgency, zeal, and purpose.

Cultivating this capacity for letting go is crucial for authentic aging because, as we get older, our identities are under continual threat. The loss of loved ones, major illnesses, children leaving home, career changes, retirement, and moving into assisted living facilities are all reminders of our own impermanence. To cope with these changes authentically, it is important to be flexible, to loosen our controlling grip on things, and to be willing to "give up" on self-interpretations that are no longer viable. Authentic resoluteness, in Heidegger's words, "discloses to existence that its uttermost possibility lies in *giving itself up*, and thus it shatters all one's tenaciousness to whatever existence one has reached."[30] But being willing to let go or give up on oneself does not mean that the choices and commitments that sustained our former selves become irrelevant. Indeed, central to the account of existence as an ongoing process of self-making is the importance of developing a sense of cohesion or unity whereby we can understand our current and future selves only insofar as this understanding coheres with our past.

This willingness to let go exposes one of the more destructive aspects of our ageist culture, one that perpetuates the view that the elderly are somehow separate and discontinuous from their younger or middle-aged selves. The stereotype assumes that there is some invisible threshold that we pass when we get older to a place where we are no longer regarded as the persons we used to be or even persons at all. "Thinking of myself as an older person when I am twenty or forty," writes Simone de Beauvoir, "means thinking of myself as *someone else*, as another than myself."[31] This points to the importance of cultivating a sense of narrative cohesion, one that can bind the various stages of one's life into a unified whole. Rather than viewing old age as an experience of fragmentation or splitting off from one's former self, the idea of coherence can illuminate the aging process as one that is continuous with the rest of one's life story.[32] But the notion of narrative cohesion is problematic for the elderly because the discursive resources or language required for self-constitution are largely ageist. Language, in this view, is best understood as a context of meaning that both expresses social realities and establishes the value and significance of those realities.[33] Given this context, the story of aging in our culture is largely about the loss of one's former self.

Yet part of what is entailed in an existential awakening is the recognition that the cultural norms and taken-for-granted truths that hold this context of meaning together are precarious and contingent. We slip into inauthenticity or self-deception when we buy into the ageist stereotypes as representative of the way things "really are." For the existentialists, this is why the anxiety provoked by the midlife crisis is so important. This anxiety has the power to shake us out of the self-deceptive prejudices of everyday life and open us up to other ways of interpreting who we are as we move into old age. As we have seen, if we are authentic and own up to the aging process, the contraction of time, and our inescapable movement toward disability and death, we can access reservoirs of depth and richness that are largely closed off to us when we are healthy and distracted by the busyness of youth. Our interpersonal communication can deepen by cutting through trivialities and gossip with honest conversations that engage the pain and vulnerability of being human. The breakdown of the body can pull us out of our harried restlessness, slowing us down and granting us access to the poignancy of the present moment. And aging can illuminate the value of ontological flexibility, of letting go of the ego and freeing ourselves from identities that are no longer livable. Indeed it could be argued that the idea of existential awakening confirms a number of recent studies that challenge the stereotype of aging, revealing the so-called "paradox of well-being."[34] The paradox is that, contrary to the overwhelmingly negative cultural image of aging, the majority of elderly adults have a positive sense of who they are and of their own well-being. There is certainly nothing romantic about aging and the breakdown of the mind and body, and self-denial and existential dishonesty can be as prevalent among the elderly as it is among any other age group. But the ageist narrative of our culture is certainly not a destiny. There remains a possibility of wisdom and deep meaning when we accept our temporal constitution, an acceptance that illuminates ways of being that are all too often closed off to the young.

Notes

1. Susie Steiner, "Top Five Regrets of the Dying," *Guardian*, February 1, 2012, https://www.theguardian.com/lifeandstyle/2012/feb/01/top-five-regrets-of-the-dying.

2. It is interesting to note that the word "ageism" wasn't coined until 1969 following the passage of the Federal Discrimination in Employment Act, which designated forty as the age when one could be subject to this kind of discrimination in the workplace. Tad Friend, "Why Ageism Never Gets Old," *New Yorker*, November 13, 2017, https://www.newyorker.com/magazine/2017/11/20/why-ageism-never-gets-old.

3. See, for example, Joann M. Montepare, "Subjective Age: Toward a Guiding Lifespan Framework," *International Journal of Behavioral Development* 33, no. 1 (January 2009): 42–46; Richard P. Eibach, Steven E. Mock, and Elizabeth A. Courtney, "Having a 'Senior Moment': Induced Aging Phenomenology, Subjective Age, and Susceptibility to Ageist Stereotypes," *Journal of Experimental Social Psychology* 46, no. 4 (July 2010): 643–49.

4. Representative works by Ernest Becker on this topic include: *The Denial of Death* (New York: Free Press, 1973) and *Escape from Evil* (New York: Free Press, 1975).

5. See, for example, Jeff Greenberg, Jeff Schimel, and Andy Martens, "Chapter 2: Ageism: Denying the Face of the Future," in *Ageism: Stereotyping and Prejudice against Older Persons*, ed. Todd D. Nelson (Cambridge, MA: MIT Press, 2002), 27–48.

6. Ibid.

7. Cf., Kevin Aho, *Heidegger's Neglect of the Body* (Albany: State University of New York Press, 2009).

8. Martin Heidegger, *The Concept of Time*, trans. William McNeill (Oxford: Blackwell, 1992), 20.

9. Martin Heidegger, *Being and Time*, trans. John Macquarrie and Edward Robinson (New York: Harper and Row, 1962), 185.

10. Heidegger, *The Concept of Time*, 14.

11. Heidegger, *Being and Time*, 216.

12. Lillian B. Rubin, *Women of a Certain Age* (New York: Harper and Row, 1979), 123, cited in Jeffrey M. Clair, David A. Karp, and William C. Yoels, *Experiencing the Life Cycle: A Social Psychology of Aging* (Springfield, IL: Thomas Books, 1993), 105.

13. Heidegger, *Being and Time*, 187–88. Emphasis in original.

14. Laura L. Cartensen, "Social and Emotional Patterns in Adulthood: Support for Socioemotional Selectivity Theory," *Psychology and Aging* 7, no. 3 (September 1992): 331–38.

15. Susan Krauss Whitbourne and Joel R. Sneed, "The Paradox of Well-Being, Identity Processes, and Stereotype Threat: Ageism and Its Potential Relationships to the Self in Later Life," in *Ageism*, ed. Todd D. Nelson.

16. Senator Richard Neuberger, quoted in Irvin D. Yalom, *Existential Psychotherapy* (New York: Basic Books, 1980), 35.

17. Martin Heidegger, *Contributions to Philosophy (From Enowning)*, trans. Parvis Emad and Kenneth Maly (Bloomington: Indiana University Press, 1999), 84.

18. Heidegger, *Being and Time*, 397–98. Emphasis in original.

19. Martin Heidegger, "Hölderlin's Hymn 'Andenken,'" *Gesamtausgabe*, vol. 52 (Frankfurt am Main: Klostermann, 1977), 163–64.

20. Martin Heidegger, *Elucidations of Hölderlin's Poetry*, trans. Keith Hoeller (Amherst, NY: Humanity Books, 2000), 153. My emphasis.

21. Martin Heidegger, *Basic Questions of Philosophy: Selected "Problems" of "Logic,"* trans. Richard Rojcewicz and André Schuwer (Bloomington: Indiana University Press, 1994), 150.

22. Martin Buber, *Eclipse of God: Studies in the Relation between Religion and Philosophy* (Princeton, NJ: Princeton University Press, 2016), 4.

23. Cited in Ram Dass, *Still Here: Embracing Aging, Changing, and Dying* (New York: Riverhead Books, 2000), 39.

24. Heidegger, "Hölderlin's Hymn 'Andenken,'" 64.

25. Whitbourne and Sneed, "The Paradox of Well-Being," 243.

26. Heidegger, *Being and Time*, 67.

27. Ibid., 276. Emphasis in original.

28. Ibid., 307.

29. See, Irvin Yalom, *Existential Psychotherapy* (New York: Being Books, 1980); Irvin Yalom, *Staring at the Sun: Overcoming the Terror of Death* (San Francisco: Jossey-Bass, 2008).

30. Heidegger, *Being and Time*, 308 (my emphasis).

31. Simone de Beauvoir, *The Coming of Age* (New York: W. W. Norton, 1996), 5.

32. Alessandro Ferrara, *Reflective Authenticity: Rethinking the Project of Modernity* (London: Routledge, 1998); Hanne Laceulle, "Aging and the Ethics of Authenticity," *Gerontologist* 58, no. 5 (September 2018): 970–78.

33. Dawson Stafford Schultz and Lydia Victoria Flasher, "Charles Taylor, Phronesis, and Medicine: Ethics and Interpretation in Illness Narrative," *Journal of Medicine and Philosophy* 36, no. 4 (August 2011): 394–409.

34. See Whitbourne and Sneed, "The Paradox of Well-Being."

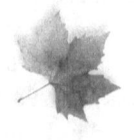

CHAPTER SIX

The End of the Story
A Narrativist View of Life's Finale

CHARLES GUIGNON

The basic facts about aging in our world are well known. In postindustrial societies over the past century, the average lifespan has increased from around fifty to nearly eighty years. It has been estimated that, by 2020, half of all humankind who have ever reached this high age will be currently alive. Commercials on television spotlight white-haired, energetic people playing with grandchildren, while a background voice sings, "Tomorrow, tomorrow." Photos of ninety-one-year-old Tony Bennett noodling with an adoring Lady Gaga headline the paper's entertainment section. And even though we agree that our contemporary world is dominated by a "youth culture," we still see politicians well on in years handling complex jobs and energetically campaigning for higher office.

Despite this omnipresence of older people in American life, there is also an uncomfortable awareness that ageism is a serious problem. The assumption that old age brings wisdom and special skills to pass on to the young has been undermined by the great leaps forward in start-up businesses and high tech typically made by younger people. Commentators point out that Larry Page and Sergey Brin were twenty-five when they started Google in 1998, whereas Mark Zuckerberg created Facebook at nineteen.[1] Ageism, the prejudice against older people that holds they are slower, duller, and less creative than young people, seems to be widespread.

This distinctively modern outlook is often contrasted with a rather romanticized vision of older age that supposedly prevailed in pre-modern cultures and may still exist elsewhere. According to this story, elders were treated as treasured reservoirs of wisdom and intuitive knowledge, a valuable segment of society to be protected and revered. Thus the Latin term for old age, which gives us our words "senescence" and "senior," was for ancient Rome the basis of the idea of a council of elders, the "Senate," which had the last word on all matters of state. Like our senators today, these older people were supposed to be accorded the highest respect and veneration.

In contrast, the now clichéd stories of Eskimos leaving their elders to die on ice floes are supported in anthropological literature with observations of tribes that buried their elders alive. An especially vivid picture of a negative view of old age comes from the Aztecs, whose warrior culture prescribed that men who turned forty-five, an age at which one was too old to fight, be given unlimited access to alcohol (a substance almost totally unknown among native peoples of the New World) so that they could drink themselves to death in a year or two.[2] The epithets still used in our world to refer to older people—"geezer," "crank," "codger," and, according to new guidelines published for journalists, even the word "elder"—show that a prejudice against old age endures into the present.

In what follows, I want to do two things. First, I want to explore insights into aging found in the mid-twentieth-century thinker Jean Améry's book *On Aging: Revolt and Resignation*, first published in 1968.[3] Améry is best known for his account of his experience in Auschwitz, but his thoughtful, existentialist-inspired book on aging remains a classic in the field. I will then turn to some themes from Heidegger's *Being and Time* to explore his account of lived time and the prospects of achieving authenticity in later life.

The Times of Our Lives

Born in Vienna in 1911, Améry first studied philosophy but then fled to Belgium when the Nazis came to power in Austria in 1938. Captured and tortured, he was sent to Auschwitz, where he survived until the fall of the Nazis. When the war was over, he returned to Brussels and became a journalist. There he wrote his most famous book, *At the Mind's Limits*, a collection of essays about Auschwitz, together with a variety of essays that made him famous. He continued to write on issues concerning mortality until 1978, when he committed suicide.

On Aging contains Améry's frequently dark reflections on the implications of existentialism for understanding the later years of life. He distinguishes three different kinds of time that may be used to characterize the stages of life. For most of a person's youth and middle years, time is experienced as a linear "lived time," the traditional conception of time as the framework for an unfolding life story. We might think of this framework as making possible a conception of life as a narrative shaped by planning and achieving goals. This mode of temporality presupposes the priority of the *future*, of what *can* and *will* be. Life is experienced as underway, a steady, cumulative movement toward the fulfillment of projects definitive of the self. As Améry points out, however, possibilities for the future are eaten away over the years so that one's identity as a self in later years comes to be defined not by one's projects but by one's possessions and past achievements. Life is contracted into what we have done and what we have.

The existentialist roots of Améry's worldview are evident in his claim, familiar to Sartreans, that the human "self," the "I" who acts and has experiences, is something that comes into existence and gets its meaning from the *look of the other*. For example, while I may swear that I feel as young as I did when I was thirty, if the eyes of others radiate back to me the perception of me as a white-haired, wrinkled, slow-moving older man, then my *self* will be what I find reflected in their eyes. The subtitle of Améry's book is therefore "*Revolt and Resignation*." The stance older people take toward this experience of being consigned to the "social time" of the *look* of others calls for an interplay of resistance and forbearance.

So I struggle against being debased to the level of "old man" or "senior citizen." But, in the end, no one ever wins this struggle against being leveled down. When we try to be "hip" or "with it" (words already loaded with yesterday's sign systems), we encounter a look that signifies "Act your age." And then the only response is a sigh that says, "Oh well." This explains Simone de Beauvoir's comment that old age "is a disqualifying process." In her words, life's "line of advance is perpetually broken by the falling back of our projects into practico-inert reality."[4] As the past expands and the future dissolves, we become, in a sense, more thinglike than human. Resistance against this fact of life seems pointless.[5]

Lived time and social time run their courses in tandem with what Améry calls "cultural time." We get a sense of what cultural time is when we begin to feel that we "do not understand the world anymore."[6] A "culture," as understood in this context, may be thought of as a significant system of symbols widely used among members of a social group at any given time. In this respect, a culture is a field of intelligibility, and being part of a culture is grasping and being competent in participating in that sign system. In Améry's view, older people often feel an aversion toward the culture of their time. They feel excluded from what they see as the "'cultural jargon' of [their] epoch."[7] Still thinking in terms of the styles common in the fifties, the older man might feel appalled when he sees young men looking scruffy, with backward baseball caps slouching around downtown. "No one dressed like that in my day," he thinks. "It looks so sloppy."

Even more broadly, the aging professor may feel that contemporary literature is no longer a pleasure to read. The absence of plot and orderly sequences of events spoils the fun of reading. He hears his young students using words like "woke" and wonders why they can't say "awakened." He complains bitterly about how difficult computers are to use, despite the fact that for decades he made no effort to master them.

No longer understanding the world, such people are dislocated from the prevailing cultural time. They have become "strangers to the world" in which they find themselves.[8] The older person may try to make the best of things—to "play along" with the new developments. But, in Améry's words, "each [person] can only become what he or she already is. The chances of transcending oneself culturally are long over with."[9] And as this becomes clearer to the older gentleman, he starts to regret "the futility of the tiresome work he put into learning about [a particular] subject" that is today considered old hat.[10] "All those years I spent trying to master Structuralism," he groans, "and today nobody even wants to hear about it."

But there is no catching up. "Even greater numbers of systems are inserting themselves, all with the effect that his own system moves further away until he scarcely recognizes it anymore. For him the logical question of whether the acceleration should be called progress is not even under discussion."[11] The upshot can be hopelessness: "The stretch of time in which we move is unkind to the aging person," writes Améry. "It is over, he has to tell himself, and it will never return again."[12]

The Possibility of Being Authentic in One's Later Years

Given the disparity among cultural interpretations of aging and the variety of individual responses that can affect the substance of a life, it might seem that nothing very general can be said about growing old. Different accounts of aging and various "how-to" books presuppose their own frames of reference—whether religious, spiritual, neoliberal, or some other. Because of this relativity of claims about aging according to a presupposed framework, sets of recommendations for living a good old age prove to be of interest only to the audiences who are already attuned to that framework. What is needed, then, is a view of aging that will speak to a wide audience because its framework is appealing to many people of different ages and backgrounds.

An attempt to satisfy this need for a very general account of the good life for humans is found in the philosopher Martin Heidegger's method of phenomenology. Following in the footsteps of Edmund Husserl, the founder of phenomenology, Heidegger sees phenomenology as a method that begins by bracketing or putting out of play the assumptions of high-level theorizing, as well as the presuppositions of our so-called common sense, in order to look at life from a fresh point of view. The goal is to show how the subjects in question—the "phenomena"—show up for us "proximally and for the most part" in "average everydayness," that is, in our pre-reflective, "average everyday" activities in a familiar lifeworld. Phenomenology in this respect is a purely descriptive methodology. It sets out to characterize how things appear to typical human beings in their ordinary lives. For our specific purposes here, I should add that people who have already entered into old age would have an advantage in this undertaking because the reality of growing older has shown up vividly in the actual course of their lives.

To get an insight into the Heideggerian view of human existence, we need to get an overview of the account of being human found in Heidegger's most influential work, *Being and Time*, first published in 1927. In this seminal work, Heidegger tries to identify what he calls "existentials," where this term refers to essential structures of human beings as these are found in familiar cases of what Heidegger calls "everydayness." The aim is to exhibit "not just any accidental [structures], but essential ones which, in every kind of Being that factical *Dasein* may possess, persist as determinative for the character of its Being."[13] The description of being human, which Heidegger refers to with the German word for "existing," *Dasein*, is supposed to capture what people are like in our most common way of being, our *Being-in-the-world*. In this technical term, the word "world" is used in the sense of a "lifeworld," as found in expressions such as "the world of theater" or "the business world." So understood, "world" refers to an intelligible context of human activities, and being-*in* a world refers to ways of being engaged in such contexts. In this view, what is basic to human existence is the fact that for us, "proximally and for the most part," to exist is to be involved in a field of meaningful connections in which equipment and practices make sense in terms of the projected outcomes of our actions.[14]

Regarded as Being-in-the world, human being is made possible by a competence we pick up in growing up into a community. The meanings that make agency and equipment intelligible to us are built into the norms we abide by from our earliest years. So, for example, I prepare classes as part of being *in* the world of academia, and I know my way around this world because it has been my professional habitat for many years.

Heidegger's description of familiar modes of human existence brings to light some of the essential structures he sees as being common to all cases of human being. One essential trait of our human being is that we are social animals. In everydayness, our Being is characterized by "*Being-with*," where this means being open to others, even when we are not actually interacting with them. The trait of *belongingness* to a wider community may take the form of mindless conformism, of just going along with the crowd, or of genuine concern. In this view, we are always receptive to others, even if such sociability takes the negative forms of disdain or hostility.[15] From this socialization, we come to master a taken-for-granted sense of what matters, or how things count—in other words, of the deep-seated values and mores of a historical culture.

Two other essential characteristics of humans shape our existence as temporal beings. On the one hand, we "always already" find ourselves *thrown* into the midst of a world, caught up in a course of events that shapes the options that are available to us. We are, in Heidegger's terminology, caught up into a world, caught up in the busyness of a public arena of life. This dimension of *situatedness* is disclosed to us by our *moods*. The German word for moods, *Stimmungen*, has the common meaning of tuning a musical instrument, and it is in this sense that, for Heidegger, *Dasein* is always in some mood or other. To say that we are always in some mood or other is to say that we are always to some extent *tuned in* to the world in some way—perhaps as anxious or bored, but always in a way that gives us an orientation toward things and others. Heidegger calls our background sense of what life is all about *facticity*.[16] It is the commonality in life forms underlying our sensitivity to moral values.

On the other hand, humans are creatures of time in the sense that they are always involved in *projecting* possibilities into the future. To be human is to be engaged in future-oriented taking a stand on the situations in which we find ourselves. Being a teacher, for example, I try to keep up with the subject I teach and look for new ways to engage my students in the material at hand. If I teach at a small college, my style and approach will be different than it would be if I taught at a state university. It is because we are temporal beings that, in Heidegger's view, we exist as *thrown projections*. I have a grasp of the norms and styles regulating the context into which I am thrown, and I naturally tend to comply with the paths dictated by those norms in taking a stand on the future. My Being is in this sense characterized by *historicity*: from the generations of teachers who preceded me, I have taken up ways of doing things that I bring to life in my own way in the classroom.[17]

The temporality of a life—this ongoing taking up of what is given in my thrownness by projecting myself toward my future—provides the basis for seeing human existence as having a narrative structure. In Heidegger's view, humans are self-constituting beings: We create our own identities through the choices we make in the contexts in which we appear on the scene. Being thrown into the world, I find myself in a situation or a set of situations that need to be addressed. By means of my actions in projecting my being toward the future, I generally follow the guidelines that give direction to our community's ways of dealing with situations of this sort. In this sense, we become the people we are in the course of enacting our life stories.

This general account of what it is to be human provides the framework for formulating some general suggestions about the character traits that make up a maximally fulfilling or "authentic" human existence. If we think of being authentic as "being true to oneself," Heidegger's general view of human life may provide some clues for envisioning an authentic way of living that we may achieve in later years. The narrative view of life assumes that how one lives one's life—one's life story as a whole—can have a *continuity* and *constancy* to the extent that the development of the story flows with evident motivation from where the story had been going so far.[18] Seen in this light, how our lives are unfolding in later years will reflect the ways they have evolved over previous years.

Heidegger suggests that one of the crucial traits of a well-lived life is *connectedness* across the life span as a whole.[19] Such cohesiveness as an aspect of life is not something that is simply given. Instead, it is something we need to strive to realize through our choices over the course of our lives. Nor is it right to think of living a coherent life as a matter of placid acceptance of what has come before. As the subtitle of Améry's book makes clear, aging almost invariably calls for a "revolt" against forces that tend to level down or deform our lives. Unexpected developments that defy incorporation into any master plot may always arise, and these developments may be hard to weave into the whole without distortion. In this respect, being true to oneself in the way called for by the ideal of "authenticity" can require considerable effort. But Heidegger holds that *steadiness* and *steadfastness* can provide connections between earlier and later events, leading to a sense of wholeness that makes life fulfilling.[20]

Heidegger's characterization of authentic existence offers a perspective on the traits that are necessary for achieving an authentic old age. A character trait that is central to being authentic at any stage of life is *resoluteness*.

In the middle years of life, being resolute can help us hold to the deepest commitments that structure our lives. It might seem unclear, however, how resoluteness can play a role in later years. Older people who try to stick to their guns can seem pig-headed or just cranky. For example, they might defy their well-intentioned mature children by holding on to quirky ways of doing things that are hopelessly out of fashion—perhaps applying layers of make-up that would be excessive even on a younger woman today. But if we take seriously the subtitle of Améry's book, the word "revolt" will stand out. A person who has made resoluteness central to her life may stick to her ways of doing things even when they seem capricious. I think there is an advantage to this sort of rebelliousness: It helps the older person to maintain a sense of independence and distinctive self-worth.

The second term in Améry's subtitle, "resignation," suggests the key concept from Heidegger's later writings, *Gelassenheit*, or "letting be." This sort of acceptance of what is, if it is not demeaning, gives the older person a way to choose reconciliation with what-is, thereby making it a matter of his or her own choice. When I lived in Japan for a while, I traveled with my host family to the countryside to visit the home of a very old gentleman called "uncle" by nearly everyone. This man lived alone, spending his time shaping tree seedlings into the miniature *bonsai* trees famous in Japan. Although well into his eighties, the uncle's eyes sparkled with pleasure. Using wires and patience, he gently pressed the branches and trunk of the miniature trees, molding them to a shape that was inherent in the nature of this particular tree and at the same time in accord with ancient traditions of making miniature trees. Laughing good-naturedly, he commented that this activity displays the struggle of humans against nature, an exercise as pointless as it is calming. He gave the trees away to anyone who showed an interest. What his activity shows is how intervening in nature can be coupled with a "letting be" that follows the natural direction of growth of the tree. The uncle clearly understood his older years as participating in the interplay between the human quest for control, on the one hand, and compliance with nature on the other.

The Japanese uncle's attitude toward nature also reveals a model of *reverence*, the gentle respect paid to nature or to noble traditions that provide us with such a productive way of passing time in the later years. Such examples of authenticity in later life show us how a well-lived life can reach its culmination with gladness and love of life and the world—*if* the way is prepared by authentic existence in earlier years. The trait of future-directedness so important to one's middle years is curtailed by the passing of time. But there is the prospect of inner peace and of gentle good humor in these ways of aging. As the Roman philosopher Cicero said more than two thousand years ago, "The course of a life cannot change. Nature has but a single path and you travel it only once. Each stage of life has its own appropriate qualities. . . . These are fruits that must be harvested in due season."[21]

Notes

1. Tad Friend, "Getting On: Why Ageism Never Gets Old," *New Yorker*, November 20, 2017, https://www.newyorker.com/magazine/2017/11/20/why-ageism-never-gets-old, 46.

2. Warwick Bray, *The Everyday Lives of the Aztecs* (New York: Hippocrene Books, 1987).

3. Jean Améry, *On Aging: Revolt and Resignation*, trans. John D. Barlow (Bloomington: Indiana University Press, 1994).

4. Simone de Beauvoir, *The Coming of Age*, trans. P. O'Brian (New York: W. W. Norton & Company), 382, 380.

5. As a rule, Dylan Thomas's "Rage, rage against the dying of the light" is not really socially acceptable. His proposal that "old age should burn and rage at the close of day" gets harder and harder to pull off as the end nears.

6. Améry, *On Aging*, 78.

7. Ibid., 78.

8. Ibid., 85.

9. Ibid., 91.

10. Ibid., 96.

11. Ibid., 96.

12. Ibid., 98.

13. Martin Heidegger, *Being and Time*, trans. John Macquarrie and Edward Robinson (New York: Harper and Row, 1962), 38.

14. Ibid., Sections 12–20.

15. Ibid., Div. I, chap. 4.

16. Ibid., Div. I, chap. 5, Sections 29–30.

17. Ibid., Div. II, chaps. 3, 4, and 5.

18. Ibid., 369. To say that continuity, steadfastness, coherence, and cohesiveness (along with other features of a well-lived life) are made possible by authenticity is not to say that anyone who exemplifies such traits is therefore authentic. Nor is there any reason to think, as students sometimes protest, that Hitler or other sociopaths might have been authentic because they've had these traits. As Somogy Varga argues, genuine authenticity requires a rich sensitivity to moral values that sociopaths lack. See Varga's *Authenticity as an Ethical Ideal* (New York: Routledge, 2012).

19. See, *inter alia*, Heidegger, 439.

20. Ibid., 369.

21. Cicero, *How to Grow Old*, trans. Philip Freeman (Princeton, NJ: Princeton University Press, 2016), 69.

CHAPTER SEVEN

Happiness and Aging
An Unlikely Combination?

BRYAN S. TURNER

There is a huge literature on happiness that stretches across every discipline.[1] However, the irony of this long history of research into happiness is that there is no satisfactory definition, let alone understanding, of this condition.[2] Within this field of research, Aristotle's analysis of happiness (as *eudaimonia* has been defined) is a constant reference. Given the lengthening life spans enjoyed by modern populations, his commentary on the nature of happiness and the conditions that promote it are especially pertinent to contemporary debates about happiness and aging. The complexity surrounding Aristotle's *eudaimonia* as a notion of human flourishing, I argue, provides a platform for criticism of the modern idea of personal happiness as contentment or "feeling good." For Aristotle, the good life and happiness were inextricably connected to the practice of virtue in a society (the polis); hence, we cannot understand human flourishing outside of political life. For Aristotle, happiness is not about pleasure or feeling good, and it would be wrong to conclude that he offers us neat, conclusive answers to puzzles about aging in modern societies. Aristotle's value is that he sets us on the right path with penetrating insights that lead to better questions.

Two Views of Aging

The legendary film star Bette Davis (1908–89) is a useful if controversial figure on which to hang two contrasting views of aging, especially the meaning and experience of the process. Diagnosed with breast cancer in 1983, she subsequently suffered four strokes that resulted in the paralysis of her left side. Continuing to smoke a hundred cigarettes a day, Davis defined the negative model in her unforgettable declaration, "Old age ain't no place for sissies." This depressing comment perhaps summarizes the conventional pessimistic view that aging is essentially a miserable experience, but Davis also saw the continuing possibility of human flourishing in aging. Thus she also asserted that "the key to life is accepting challenges. Once someone stops doing this, he's dead." This alternative vision captures the contemporary, more optimistic view of aging as an open challenge that can result in positive experiences. The optimistic view prevails in contemporary gerontology, but often at the cost of translating "happiness" as merely emotional contentment.

One might assume that sociologists would be at the forefront of this research, but, with a few exceptions, such as Amitai Etzioni, they have not engaged with the issue; happiness research, consequently, is largely dominated by psychologists, economists, and historians.[3] Another exception in sociology is Alasdair MacIntyre, insofar as he argues, in *After Virtue: A Study of Moral Theory* (1984), that Max Weber provides the only cogent description of modernity.[4] In his engagement with Aristotle, MacIntyre has emerged as the primary critic of emotivism in a society in which others are simply means to satisfy one's ends and values are justified by subjective preference. For the modern consumer, happiness is disconnected from everyday experiences of social belonging and political life more broadly when being happy is defined and promoted by corporations in the interest of selling goods and services that, we are told, will make us feel good as private individuals. Critics of Aristotle have argued that the difference between the Aristotelian concept of *eudaimonia* and modern notions of happiness is that, whereas Aristotle's approach is "objective" and "stringent," the modern version is "subjective" and "flexible."[5] However, my argument is more nearly that, for Aristotle, whether or not individuals flourish is a political issue. In short, the Aristotelian legacy confronts psychological indexes of happiness by insisting on the political context of human flourishing. A similar criticism of the subjective well-being model has been developed by Richard Ryan and Edward Deci in their contrast between the modern "hedonic" approach of psychology and the eudaimonic approach of Aristotelian philosophy.[6]

One other important lesson from this Aristotelian legacy is that happiness does not have a continuous history. For example, we can discern an important shift in visions of the human condition taking place in the late nineteenth and early twentieth centuries. Following the demise of utilitarianism, the period 1890–1930 ushered in a pessimistic rejection of the goal of happiness. For thinkers ranging from Nietzsche to Freud, happiness had become an illusion. Benedetto Croce said of his generation that its members, unlike the Greeks, no longer believed in the prospect of happiness in this world or in the Christian church's promise of otherworldly happiness.[7] It is perhaps not surprising that for MacIntyre, any description of the modern world comes down to a choice between the romantic Nietzsche and the analytical Weber.

If the final decades of the nineteenth century induced a melancholy view of reality, the predominant perspective on happiness and aging since the 1970s has been overwhelmingly positive. In the United Kingdom, a view of aging as entering a period of creativity was described by Peter Laslett in his 1991 book *A Fresh Map of Life: The Emergence of the Third Age*.[8] Contemporary approaches sustain this upbeat account. This trend is illustrated by the psychological research into aging and happiness by Laura Carstensen and Steven Pinker's defense of the Enlightenment, as well as Pinker's claims that modern societies are more peaceful than those of the past and that progress toward greater human happiness is occurring concurrently with economic progress.[9]

Although in the present chapter I am mainly concerned with debates about happiness in the humanities and social sciences, the optimistic view of successful aging cannot be separated from advances in medical science, especially in biotechnology. Aubrey de Grey and his colleagues advance the view that human well-being is now underpinned by advances in science. Thus, given time and investment, modern medicine will be able to eliminate the chronic conditions that attend aging. In other words, the prospect exists that we can live forever. In their 2008 book *Ending Aging*, de Grey and coauthor Michael Rae treat aging as merely an engineering problem, promoting the idea of eradicating death through what they call "Strategies for Engineered Negligible Senescence," or SENS.[10]

Though recent developments in microbiology and related technologies are framed as offering a promise of living forever, there are, in principle, three possible outcomes: a relatively long life, but with many forms of disability and immobility; an extension of life, with a quick death as a conclusion; or delayed or deferred death. While these outcomes might look more like survival than living, de Grey also argues that the existing range of psychological problems associated with aging—depression, anxiety, boredom, and despair—could be remediated by a variety of drugs. This dream of longevity, youthfulness, and happiness has to be taken seriously in part because considerable investment has already been made in the longevity project. However, de Grey and his colleagues have been charged with understating the social costs and risks of indefinite life prolongation.[11] Survival may, in fact, incur the curse of "a new age of extended debility."[12]

My overall criticism of aging research is that both optimists and pessimists, while researching emotions, cognitive processes, memory, or contentment, tend to neglect our embodiment, and hence ignore the less dramatic experiences of everyday discomfort. Aubrey de Grey, in my estimation, treats longevity as mere survival, in which unhappiness could be treated, I assume, with psychedelic drugs. Aging research needs the sociology of the body, which takes account of our shared vulnerability and exposure to creeping disability and immobility.[13]

Happiness in Aristotle's Nicomachean Ethics *and the* Politics

We should note at the outset that *eudaimonia* is somewhat misleadingly translated as "happiness," whereas Aristotle is more exactly concerned with well-being or flourishing. In *The Fragility of Goodness*, Martha Nussbaum neatly summarized the essence of Greek ethics, which involved "the aspiration to rational self-sufficiency."[14] In turn, this aim meant that the contingency of life or the role of luck and the vulnerability of humans were fundamental challenges to the quest for a virtuous life and self-sufficiency. Happiness was to be thought of as activity directed toward the good life. On this basis, Nussbaum is also critical of the translation of *eudaimonia* that would connect it with modern ideas about pleasure. She writes that, given the heritage of Kantian ethics and utilitarianism, modern thinkers treat happiness as "the name of a feeling of contentment or pleasure, and a view that gives supreme value to psychological states rather than to activities. . . . To the Greeks *eudaimonia* means something like 'living a good life for a human being.'"[15] We might also give a somewhat different slant on the idea of fragility by connecting it to the idea of our bodily vulnerability under three observations: We are vulnerable with respect to (a) our physical and cultural inheritance at birth, (b) our constant exposure to accidents and mishaps, and (c) the eventual breakdown of our bodies.

To understand Aristotle's argument, we need to understand his basic problem, namely, identifying the *ergon* ("function") of human beings, since it is the *ergon* that makes a thing what it is.[16] The true *ergon* of humans is the measure of human excellence, and it defines us as human rather than something else. But what separates us from the animals? We share with them basic bodily needs. (We should note that Aristotle is fully aware of the fact that in terms of sleep, nutrition, and sexual intercourse, nothing separates us from the animal world.) It is, rather, how we use (or misuse) our bodies that gives rise to moral praise or condemnation. Our happiness, the ultimate aim of all human life, is connected to purposeful activity directed at well-being. Through consideration of the *ergon* of the human being—"activity of soul in accord with reason"—three criteria emerge for the highest good: being (a) complete or final, (b) self-sufficient, and (c) choice-worthy.[17] By applying these criteria, Aristotle arrives, in the *Nicomachean Ethics*, at the preliminary definition of *eudaimonia* as "an activity of soul in accord with virtue" (I.7, 1098a17). He further analyzes the issue by taking up the question of how *eudaimonia* is related to "external goods" and chance. Before moving on to a thorough analysis of various individual virtues, he concludes the first book of the *Ethics* with the understanding that, while the virtuous person is not beholden to chance, his happiness might be.

While giving a final and settled definition of happiness, Aristotle is clearer in his mind as to what happiness is not. He rejects a number of popular accounts of happiness: "The many and crudest seem to suppose, not unreasonably, that the good and happiness are pleasure" (I.5, 1095b15–16). "The refined and active, on the other hand, choose honor" (I.5, 1095b22–23). After further discussion, he finally rejects popular ideas that happiness is pleasure, wealth, and honor. His purpose is to show how happiness is chosen as an end in and for itself. Having rejected many possibilities, Aristotle proposes his definition of happiness (*eudaimonia*) as connected to virtue. If happiness is conjoined with virtue, how is it obtained? It is a matter of habituation in virtue, and hence, through experience, people gain wisdom and are more likely to make rational choices. Indeed, we should not leave happiness to chance, for no matter how much education and virtue we enjoy, we may experience calamities and disasters. Trials and tribulations of life can always strike the most virtuous.

This is the opening account, then, of Aristotle's ethics in Book I, where we have seen that he makes the basic claim that happiness is "a certain activity of soul in accord with complete virtue" (I.13, 1102a5–6). However, he has already identified certain problems that persist in his account here and in other works. One basic problem is that he wants to treat happiness as in some way whole, complete, and final. He does not want to think that we can be a little bit happy one day and very unhappy the next. Happiness is final because it is an activity of the soul. A man who is happy should not be so easily blown off course by small misfortunes. The obvious question, therefore, is whether we can call a person truly happy only at the end of his life.

While Aristotle has been somewhat successful in rejecting pleasure, honor, and money as equivalents of happiness, his final answer as to what it is illustrates the problems that have never been adequately resolved in contemporary approaches. He is troubled by the notion that acquiring happiness is simply a matter of chance or luck. If we possess happiness thanks merely to the lucky accident of good health or wealthy and influential parents, happiness cannot carry the ethical weight he wants to attach to it. Alternatively, he thinks that happiness cannot be entirely the product of personal striving and education. If it were, we could praise people simply for being happy. "Indeed," he writes, "praise belongs to virtue: people are apt to do noble things as a result of virtue" (I.12, 1101b32–33).

In Book I of the *Politics*, Aristotle ultimately concludes that happiness is divine in origin, a gift of the gods. As the Greeks of Aristotle's time used it, *eudaimonia* literally meant being possessed of a benevolent demon or spirit. The term itself perhaps misleadingly suggests a role for the chance intervention of the gods or for good fortune in personal happiness. The other interesting aspect of Aristotle's reflections is that, especially in the *Politics*, he argues that *eudaimonia* can also be an attribute of the state—the polis can flourish just as humans can, or not. Indeed, for Aristotle the two are linked: Citizens flourish (i.e., are happy) in states that are flourishing (i.e., are happy states). In Book III of the *Politics*, he argues that "Living well, then, is the end of the city. . . . A city is the community of families and villages in a complete and self-sufficient life. This, we assert, is living happily and finely."[18]

Aristotle recognized that, while everybody wants happiness, there is no agreement on what it is. There is, however, an important difference between our understanding of happiness and the *eudaimonia* of the Greek world. While happiness for the ancients was bound up with the collective experience of good government, contemporary notions of happiness are typically individualistic, tending to confuse pleasure with happiness. For example, Christian Smith's survey of young adults in the United States found that they associate personal happiness with consumption and that their dominant aim in life "is to have the financial means to possess and consume material goods, enjoyable services and fulfilling experiences."[19] However, as we shall see, for writers like Steven Pinker, the consumption of material goods, enjoyment of efficient services, and experience of fulfilling activities *are* happiness.

The message of the *Nicomachean Ethics* is that happiness requires a virtuous life, and such a life is premised on our personal autonomy, namely, our control over our lives and our capacity to make rational decisions. This notion of self-sufficiency, or "the aspiration to rational self-sufficiency," is not especially innocent in Aristotle's account.[20] To have happiness, we have to have personal autonomy, and that excludes slaves, workers, women, and, toward the end of their lives, the elderly, from achieving happiness. For Aristotle, aging is a process whereby we lose our self-sufficiency and autonomy and, as a result, enter into a type of slavery not as the property of another but simply as a consequence of physical decline. However, this process somewhat contradicts the idea that we are happy because we are virtuous. With aging, we are unhappy as a consequence of the loss of physical vitality rather than through a loss of virtue.

Aristotle and the Disengagement Theory

Having broadly described *eudaimonia*, I will now turn in more detail to Aristotle's view of old age and to some of the puzzles that remain in his work and his legacy. Despite the difficulties of translation and interpretation, Aristotle's idea of well-being is certainly relevant to any understanding of aging and happiness. However, there is only a limited discussion of aging in the *Nicomachean Ethics*. On the one hand, in Book IX Aristotle reflects on intergenerational responsibilities and says, "To every old man is due the honor that accords with age, in rising and giving him a seat at the table and such things" (IX.2, 1165a27–29). On the other hand, he also has some negative things to say, for instance, "Stinginess is both incurable (for it seems that age and every infirmity make people stingy) and inborn in human beings to a greater degree than is prodigality" (IV.1, 1121b13–15). He also considers whether we can call somebody happy before that person's life is complete: "Many reversals and all manner of fortune arise in the course of life, and it is possible for someone who is particularly thriving to encounter great disasters in old age, just as the myth is told about Priam in the Trojan tales. Nobody deems happy someone who deals with fortune of that sort and comes to a wretched end" (I.9, 1100a5–9). In *On Rhetoric*, he suggests that while the young live in hope, the old live in memory, because their futures hold limited years.[21] Toward the end of life our activities are constrained, and we cannot enjoy the self-sufficiency Aristotle considers essential to *eudaimonia*.

Howard H. Harriot captures what has been seen as Aristotle's negative view of aging. According to Harriot, it has

> survived antiquity, Renaissance thinking, and Romanticism, and it manifests itself in the assumptions of disengagement theory. The general view is that outside the world of work (which Josiah Royce, for example, tied to the answer to the question of what "personhood" con-

sists of), the inference can be drawn that in old age one ceases to satisfy the condition of full personhood, since this is often tied to a partial disengagement from the world, and "personhood" is itself defined by the existence of projects which the person is trying to realize, often within the constraints of a working life (career).[22]

For Aristotle, the loss of vitality in old age is a result of the loss of *thumos* (or *thymos*), namely "spiritedness" that involves emotions, desires, and passions. For instance, a strong, youthful stallion has *thumos*. Its loss involves a related process of loss of *epithumia*, or appetite or affection. (A slight variant on this word, *epithumeo*, is also used to describe any desire for something). The loss of *thumos* is a physical process that, Aristotle observes, is inevitable in old age. This is one reason that Aristotle's critics often connect his legacy to the theory of aging as disengagement.[23] Cumming and Henry describe aging as involving an "inevitable mutual withdrawal or disengagement resulting in decreased interaction between the aging person and others in the social system to which they belong."[24]

Is Aristotle's approach to aging a version of disengagement theory? Perhaps his own life experience offers a clue to his philosophy here. What we do know suggests that he died at what was, for his society, an extremely old age, 62 years. It is perhaps ironic that, because of political problems following the death of Alexander the Great in 323 BC, Aristotle died in exile as a consequence of a digestive disease. We cannot completely grasp Aristotle's theory of aging without some insight into the demographics of his time and place and without situating his interpretation of happiness in a political framework. Aristotle's own "disengagement" was itself a consequence of political instability.

While most discussions of Aristotle on happiness focus on the *Ethics*, we cannot ignore the *Politics*, in which happiness has a thoroughly political emphasis that illuminates the contrast between his view of the good life and modern discussions of happiness (and aging) as more psychological than political. Happy, successful citizens were an inseparable component of a successful polis. Good government was necessary for good living. The causes of happiness are complex and controversial, but there is a consensus that wealth is not necessarily decisive. Generally speaking, people in poor countries in Latin America are as happy as, or even happier than, people in wealthy developed societies. The main point here is to contrast Aristotle's view of *eudaimonia*, in which a happy and flourishing polis is a necessary condition for happy and flourishing citizens, with contemporary research in which, while there is much talk about happiness, it is largely understood as an individual and passive experience associated with pleasure (especially the pleasure of privatized consumption). Although, as we have seen, there are many problems with Aristotle's vision, he makes a serious attempt to define happiness beyond simple notions of individual feelings of satisfaction or pleasure. The conditions of happiness are ultimately political and social.

Old Age and Happiness

Stephen Pinker's book *Enlightenment Now*, which includes a chapter on happiness, is an influential example of the contemporary and more optimistic picture of aging and old age.[25] Pinker is primarily interested in the comparative relationships between wealth and happiness. The basic argument is simple enough. Generally speaking, modern societies are getting richer, and rich people and rich societies are happier than poor people and poor societies. Pinker argues that while there are important variations within and between countries, in global terms happiness has increased: "We know that richer people within a country are happier, that richer countries are happier, and that people get happier as their countries get richer (which means that people get happier over time)."[26] He believes that the facts speak for themselves, and thus he draws on multiple sources to show that people are living longer and that they become happier as they age.

Pinker recognizes many of the methodological problems that arise when historical and comparative judgments are made about happiness. It makes a big difference whether we are talking about changes across the life cycle, the historical period, or multiple generations. He also recognizes that there are ups and downs in happiness. Unsurprisingly the Great Depression "left a scar on the generations who came of age as it deepened."[27] In a general observation about aging, Pinker writes that "people tend to get happier as they get older (an age effect), presumably because they overcome the hurdles of embarking on adulthood and develop the wisdom to cope with setbacks and to put their lives in perspective. (They may pass through a midlife crisis on the way, or take a final slide in the last years of old age.)"[28]

While I am critical of Pinker's perspectives on age and aging, I will start by saying that I am sympathetic to his view that modern history cannot be written off as an abysmal failure, and I have argued in an article on happiness and successful societies that sociology is a modern dismal science that competes with economics to give a depressing, Malthusian view of the world.[29] Pinker's challenge and his methodology (just count!) cannot be easily ignored, because demography is to a large degree on his side. We are living longer lives that are supported by dramatic advances in medical science. In global terms, total fertility rates have fallen dramatically, leaving women with better health and enhanced opportunities to participate outside the domestic sphere. I, too, want to see success and improvement, but I am critical of Pinker's account of age and aging. So what are the problems with his (and other optimistic) views of aging and the aging experience?

For one, Pinker never really defines happiness. He believes it exists if people say they are happy. For Aristotle, being happy because of good fortune would have made his attempts to connect happiness (flourishing) with virtue or living an honorable life unsatisfactory. Instead, Aristotle connects living well with virtue in a flourishing society. A virtuous person can withstand the tribulations of mere fortune. In Pinker's account, if people say they are happy in response to survey questionnaires, then they are happy. In other words, his largely implicit definition equates feelings of contentment with happiness. Therefore, happiness has ceased to be the ultimate goal of human endeavor and is now conceptualized as contentment arising from the material improvement of society.

My second criticism is that there are no bodies in Pinker's view of aging. Apparently old people are happy even in the company of creaking joints, incontinence, digestive problems, skin irritations, and muscle loss. One might reasonably argue that modern medicine, especially palliative care, has been very successful at eliminating pain, but it has had less success eliminating the everyday discomforts of aging. The management of chronic pain among the elderly is increasingly associated with drug dependency. However, I recognize that one has to be careful with such arguments. Pain may present itself and be experienced in different ways across different cultures, as Margaret Lock demonstrated in her ethnographic study of the experience and meaning of menopause in North America and Japan.[30] Lock proposes that "local biologies" have to be understood in terms of their distinctive cultural settings. This research should not, of course, obscure the fact that American and Japanese women go through menopause and experience aging by virtue of having bodies.

How does Pinker depart from Aristotle? He believes that modern happiness is no longer connected to virtue or to any collective experience of citizenship. Although he quotes economic data on wealth as a source of modern happiness, his actual explanations tend to be psychological rather than economic. He pays little attention to the changing political and communal aspects of the quest for happiness.

In order to understand individual aging and happiness, we need to consider the wider social and political context of well-being. For example, research emerging in the United States about addiction and its impact on life expectancy may undermine Pinker's overall optimism about social change. An opioid crisis started in the United States in the 1990s that has continued to intensify. The National Institute on Drug Abuse reported that in 2016 over 64,000 Americans died from drug overdoses, 21 percent more than in 2015.[31] Opioids were the cause of about 34,000 of these deaths. Pinker makes brief reference to the opioid epidemic in which he attempts to show that the generation born between 1953 and 1963 is the most affected by addiction. Hence, he characterizes the present crisis as "an epidemic of the druggy Baby Boomers cohort reaching middle age."[32] This interpretation is simplistic. Opioid addiction now afflicts all age groups (not just "druggy Baby Boomers"), and though the five most affected states are West Virginia, New Hampshire, Kentucky, Ohio, and Rhode Island, it has become a problem throughout the United States. As much as 40 percent of older adults suffer chronic pain, a condition for which they are routinely treated with opioids.[33] The makeup of these drugs themselves is changing with the spread of fentanyl, a synthetic opioid that is trafficked out of Mexico. Given the absence of adequate treatment centers and an effective national policy, there are no easy solutions to the epidemic, which brings into question Pinker's blanket optimism.[34]

Although Pinker's evolutionary optimism about happiness has been criticized, there is considerable social-psychological research that gives some empirical support to his views. Much of this empirical work has been the result of investigations by Laura Carstensen and her colleagues, primarily from the Stanford Center on Longevity in Palo Alto, California. Carstensen and colleagues have done much to reconcile the paradox of, on the one hand, ample evidence of decreased biological, physiological, and cognitive capacity and, on the other, empirical findings that in old age people experience generally high levels of well-being. Carstensen and a fellow investigator, Margret Baltes, have argued that an understanding of adaptive aging resolves the paradox by offering a better understanding of resilience in the aging process.[35] According to this research, the elderly are selective in the retention of good and bad memories of the past. Screening out negative experiences makes life appear to be rewarding despite the physical and mental decline that accompanies aging.[36] Carstensen's book *A Long Bright Future* offers a popular version of solid empirical research into aging over two decades.[37]

Carstensen's work basically covers aging in terms of the themes of adaptation, emotional life and aging, and our understanding of time. She recognizes that aging involves a decline in cognitive processing, but she claims that the subjective experience of normal aging is generally positive.[38] Most of the objective measures available indicate that older citizens continue to be involved in families and communities. Their emotional well-being is at least as good as that of members of younger age groups. Older people feel more satisfied with their social relationships, especially with their own children. The paradox of aging—cognitive decline coexistent with emotional well-being—is associated with the horizon of time. Because older people perceive time as constrained rather than limitless, they concentrate on emotional satisfaction. Older people are selective about what can give them this satisfaction. Carstensen also found from experiments with a cohort of nuns that there is a tendency for aspects of personal biography to be more positively evaluated; she also found that accumulated positive memories facilitate adaptive aging.

Carstensen's research finds further support in psychological studies that nevertheless find that improvements in individual well-being can never be isolated from improvements in the social environment. Thus, for example, different cohorts will exhibit improvements in cognitive function, "presumably due to culture-based advances in the course of the past century" and the fact that historical trends that favor later generations "carry into old age [and] constitute strong effects at age 75."[39]

Happiness in Old Age

Returning to my opening reference to Bette Davis, she implicitly noted that our notions of happiness are never stable: they are perceived as either misery or opportunity. In the modern period, we have seen a remarkable return to the idea that happiness is not only desirable but available even in old age. Unsurprisingly, this contemporary optimism takes various forms: Pinker's evolutionary Enlightenment, Carstensen's psychology of emotions, and de Grey's utopia of endless existence. I have criticized this post-Aristotelian world because happiness has become almost entirely a subjective feeling of contentment divorced from its location in politics and civil society. Long life cannot be easily distinguished from mere survival into old age, and it is doubtful that modern medicine alone, despite its spectacular advances, can deliver a long life for everybody. We must not confuse living successfully with merely surviving, which in itself has little moral justification and is largely devoid of meaning.

As I have argued through much of my academic career, the human body is strangely absent in the social sciences and is underrepresented even in medical sociology.[40] Much of the research I have considered in the present chapter fails to give sufficient attention to the actual character of embodiment in old age. We cannot expect to sail through our lives free from the discomforts and perturbations of an aging body while at the same time claiming subjectively to be "happy." Only with an increasing dependence on pain management with modern painkillers can we hope to avoid the physical aspects of discomfort and despair. Under any set of social arrangements, aging will be a challenging experience for the great majority.

Finally, there is an opportunity here to connect Aristotle's view with a more promising view of the elderly and aging. The elderly are often seen as repositories of wisdom as a consequence of the challenges we all face in the life course. Aristotle, for instance, did recognize that "one ought to pay attention to the undemonstrated assertions and opinions of experienced and older people, or of the prudent, no less than to demonstrations, for because they have an experienced eye, they see correctly" (VI.11, 1143b11–14). This view of aging suggests that practical wisdom is a consequence of habituation over time and through the life cycle. Through habituation in virtue, a person can achieve some degree of autarchy despite the physical infirmities of aging. Subjective perceptions of control among the elderly appear to predict better physical health and memory.[41] Physical aging may in this sense find compensation in an individual's perception of control resulting in some degree of autonomy, which for Aristotle is an important condition of well-being. Aristotle may have been prejudiced in believing that the elderly are invariably disagreeable and prone to meanness (*Nicomachean Ethics*, IV.1, 1121b13–14). However, Donnellan and Lucas found that older adults can manage interpersonal problems more effectively than young adults because they have more experience dealing with adversity and better control over their emotions.[42] These findings from psychology are consistent with Pinker's view that the elderly have the wisdom to cope with personal troubles.

Despite the technological advances in contemporary societies that inevitably create an enormous difference between us moderns and the ancients, Aristotle helps us to bring several crucial ideas into any conception of a good life in old age: attention to our vulnerability and embodiment, virtue, the political community, and training to overcome bad luck. Despite the technological advances, we share with Aristotle the same limitations and potentialities as arise from a shared embodiment—aging being the most significant.

Notes

1. Darrin M. McMahon, *Happiness: A History* (New York: Grove Press, 2006).

2. Bryan S. Turner and Yuri Contreras-Vejar, "Happiness," *The Wiley Blackwell Encyclopedia of Social Theory*, ed. Bryan S. Turner, vol. 3 (Hoboken, NJ: Wiley, 2018), 1030–37.

3. For an example of his sociological work on happiness, see Amitai Etzioni, "Happiness Is the Wrong Metric," *Society* 53, no. 3 (April 2016): 246–57.

4. Alasdair MacIntyre, *After Virtue: A Study in Moral Theory* (Notre Dame, IN: University of Notre Dame Press, 1984), 109.

5. See, for example, Richard Kraut, "Two Conceptions of Happiness," *Philosophical Review* 88, no. 2 (April 1979): 167–97.

6. Richard M. Ryan and Edward L. Deci, "On Happiness and Human Potentials: A Review of Research on Hedonic and Eudaimonic Well-Being," *Annual Review of Psychology* 52, no. 1 (February 2001): 141–66.

7. Benedetto Croce, cited in H. Stuart Hughes, *Consciousness and Society: The Reorientation of Social Thought, 1890–1930* (London: MacGibbon and Kee, 1959), 428.

8. Peter Laslett, *A Fresh Map of Life: The Emergence of the Third Age* (Boston: Harvard University Press, 1991).

9. For Laura L. Carstensen's work on aging and happiness, see, "Selectivity Theory: Social Activity in Life-Span Context," *Annual Review of Gerontology and Geriatrics* 11 (1991): 195–217; "Social and Emotional Patterns in Adulthood: Support for Socioemotional Selectivity Theory," *Psychology and Aging* 7, no. 3 (September 1992), 331–38; and *A Long Bright Future* (New York: Broadway Books, 2009). For Steven Pinker's defense of the Enlightenment and research on happiness, see *The Better Angels of Our Nature: Why Violence Has Declined* (New York: Penguin, 2011), and *Enlightenment Now: The Case for Reason, Science, Humanism, and Progress* (London: Allen Lane, 2018).

10. Aubrey de Grey and Michael Rae, *Ending Aging: The Rejuvenation Breakthrough That Could Reverse Human Aging in Our Lifetime* (London: St. Martin's Press, 2008).

11. See Daniel Callahan, "Life Extension: Rolling the Technological Dice," *Society* 46, no. 3 (May 2009): 214–20.

12. Eric Cohen, "The Phenomenon of Death," *Society* 46, no. 3 (May 2009): 221–23, 221.

13. Bryan S. Turner, "The End(s) of Humanity and the Metaphors of Modernity," *Hedgehog Review* 3, no. 2 (2001): 7–32.

14. Martha C. Nussbaum, *The Fragility of Goodness: Luck and Ethics in Greek Tragedy and Philosophy*, rev. ed. (New York: Cambridge University Press, 2001), 3.

15. Ibid., 6.

16. Thomas Nagel, "Aristotle on Eudaimonia," *Phronesis* 17, no. 3 (1972): 252–59.

17. Aristotle, *The Nicomachean Ethics*, trans. Robert C. Bartlett and Susan D. Collins (Chicago: University of Chicago Press, 2011), I.7, 1098a7. Further citations of the *Nicomachean Ethics* are given by in-text parenthetical line numbers.

18. Aristotle, *Politics,* trans. Carnes Lord (Chicago: University of Chicago Press, 2013), III.9, 1280b38–42.

19. Christian Smith, *Lost in Translation: The Dark Side of Emerging Adulthood* (New York: Oxford University Press, 2011), 107.

20. Nussbaum, *The Fragility of Goodness*, 3.

21. Aristotle, *On Rhetoric: A Theory of Civic Discourse*, trans. George A. Kennedy (New York: Oxford University Press, 1991).

22. Howard H. Harriot, "Old Age, Successful Ageing and the Problem of Significance," *Ethical Perspectives* 13, no. 1 (2003): 119–43, 121. There are, of course, alternative views. Historians have generally believed that in more traditional societies old age is respected. Cowgill and Holmes have argued that modernization results in a decline in the status of the elderly in societies where innovation and change are emphasized over tradition and stability. See Donald O. Cowgill and Lowell D. Holmes, *Aging and Modernization* (New York: Appleton-Century-Crofts, 1972).

23. This critique is formulated by Elaine Cumming and William Earl Henry in *Growing Old: The Process of Disengagement* (New York: Arno, 1961).

24. Cumming and Henry, *Growing Old*, 227.

25. Ibid.

26. Ibid., 270–71.

27. Ibid., 273.

28. Ibid., 273.

29. Bryan S. Turner, "(I Can't Get No) Satisfaction: Happiness and Successful Societies," *Journal of Sociology* 54, no. 3 (2018): 279–93.

30. Margaret Lock, *Encounters with Aging: Mythologies of Menopause in Japan and North America* (Berkeley: University of California Press, 1993).

31. National Institute on Drug Abuse, "Overdose Death Rates," 2017, https://www.drugabuse.gov/related-topics/trends-statistics/overdose-death-rates.

32. Pinker, *Enlightenment Now*, 184.

33. Nora D. Volkow and A. Thomas McLellan, "Opioid Abuse in Chronic Pain—Misconception and Mitigation Strategies," *New England Journal of Medicine* 374 (March 2016): 1253–63.

34. Nabarun Dasgupta, Leo Beletsky, and Daniel Ciccarone, "Opioid Crisis: No Easy Fix to Its Social and Economic Determinants," *American Journal of Public Health* 108, no. 2 (February 2018): 182–86.

35. Margret M. Baltes and Laura L. Carstensen, "The Process of Successful Ageing," *Ageing and Society* 16 (1996): 397–422.

36. Laura L. Carstensen, Helene H. Fung, and Susan T. Charles, "Socioemotional Selectivity Theory in the Second Half of Life," *Motivation and Emotion* 7, no. 2 (2003): 103–23; Laura L. Carstensen, "Social and Emotional Patterns in Adulthood: Support for Socioemotional Selectivity Theory," *Psychology and Aging* 7, no. 3 (September 1992), 331–38.

37. Laura L. Carstensen, *A Long Bright Future* (New York: Broadway Books, 2009).

38. Susan Charles and Laura L. Carstensen, "Social and Emotional Aging," *Annual Review of Psychology* 61 (2010): 383–409.

39. Denis Gerstorf, Peter Eibich, Ilja Demuth, Elisabeth Steinhagen-Thiessen, Gizem Hülür, Johanna Drewelies, Sandra Duezel, Paolo Ghisletta, and Gert G. Wagner, "Secular Changes in Late-Life Cognition and Well-Being: Towards a Long Bright Future with a Short Brisk Ending?," *Psychology and Aging* 30, no. 2 (2015): 301–10, 308–9.

40. Bryan S. Turner, *The Body and Society: Explorations in Social Theory* (Oxford: Blackwell, 1984).

41. Frank J. Infurna and Denis Gerstorf, "Linking Perceived Control, Physical Activity, and Biological Health to Memory Change," *Psychology and Aging* 28, no. 4 (December 2013): 1147–63; Frank J. Infurna and Denis Gerstorf, "Perceived Control Relates to Better Functional Health and Lower Cardio-Metabolic Risk: The Mediating Role of Physical Activity," *Health Psychology* 33, no. 1 (January 2014): 85–94.

42. M. Brent Donnellan and Richard E. Lucas, "Age Differences in the Big Five across the Life Span: Evidence from Two National Samples," *Psychology and Aging* 23, no. 3 (September 2008): 558–66. The Big Five refers to a list of the personality traits that some believe humans display.

PART III

An Old Age That Goes Well

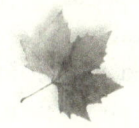

CHAPTER EIGHT

Friendship, Citizenship, and Abandonment
Older Adults with Dementia and without Family Caregivers

JANELLE S. TAYLOR

As Joseph Davis notes in the introduction to this volume, "Our cultural impoverishment is rooted, most fundamentally, in a deficient conception of the person in society." This has particularly painful consequences when aging entails, as it so often does, the development of dementia, which erodes precisely those capacities for language, memory, and cognition that are widely framed as constitutive of individual identity and necessary for relationships. As noted in an analysis published nearly two decades ago: "While 'loss of identity' or 'loss of self' is not part of the DSM-IV or any other clinical criteria for Alzheimer's disease... this popular cultural idiom is seamlessly combined with biomedical understandings. It has become part of a popular discourse of Alzheimer's . . . that imposes a kind of 'social death' on the afflicted person."[1] The losses in functioning that inevitably follow from biological processes affecting the brain are, in other words, painfully compounded when claims to social and political "recognition" are made contingent on the narrowly cognitive ability to "recognize" people, words, and things.[2]

Like many people, I have had to struggle to understand dementia because of how it landed in my life, as the daughter of a woman who lived with progressive dementia for about twenty years. I will say, however, that the same aspects of dementia that render it so personally devastating also make it anthropologically quite interesting. Dementia raises profound questions about, precisely, "the person in society." What is a person? And what qualities or capabilities are necessary for a person to be "in society"?

My own interest, over the past decade or so, has been to push back against narrow, individualistic, and biologically oriented visions of personhood and aging by seeking to document how life can be good—or at least, can be made better—even when dementia is present. To do so, I have (following the lead of many other scholars) argued for a *relational* understanding of personhood: The argument is that we may need to stop looking only to individuals as the bearers of "selfhood" and start looking more at how "selfhood" is distributed among networks, sustained by supportive environments, and emergent within practices of care.

Dementia and the Limits of Family

Where, then, do we locate this supportive environment, this network of relations, that will sustain personhood when dementia has rendered it tenuous? One obvious place to look, it might seem, would be among the same people who provide other forms of care and support.

All human beings need care, of course, but the question of who will provide it is particularly urgent for older adults with dementia. As their condition progresses, individuals living with dementia face increasing difficulties managing basic daily self-care and routine tasks without help from others (though they may not admit to needing help, or accept it when offered). Many people with dementia also have other chronic conditions, including vision, hearing, and mobility limitations, adding significantly to their levels of disability and to the complexity of the care needed to keep them in the best possible health.[3] As a consequence, their need for medical care may be great, but without assistance people living with dementia may be unable to manage the scheduling and transportation involved in doctor visits, not to mention the complex work of following medically advised regimens.[4]

Broader changes in the organization and provision of medical care have also made informal (i.e., unpaid) caregivers more necessary than ever, as the formal healthcare system delegates to them increasingly more complex and daunting tasks for which they may have received little training.[5] This is especially true at the end of life, when dementia is most common; in the United States, fewer patients are now dying in hospitals, and much of the care previously provided there has shifted to homes.[6] In this country, informal caregivers of older adults also act as geriatric case managers, medical record keepers, paramedics, and patient advocates to fill dangerous gaps in the formal healthcare system.[7] And we know that older adults who are without needed care and support suffer consequences that include falls, hospitalizations, and emergency room visits, as well as discomfort, going hungry, losing weight, dehydration, and burns.[8]

It is generally assumed (by clinicians, policymakers, and researchers, no less than by members of the public) that when an older adult needs assistance, the role of informal caregiver will be assumed by family members—and in fact that is the most common arrangement in North America. The majority of informal caregivers are adult children (most often daughters) or spouses (most often wives). The difficulties, health impacts, and economic costs that such informal caregiving exacts are well documented, and a number of policy recommendations have been proposed to better support family caregivers and attend to their needs.[9]

Well justified though they may be, the implementation of such policies still seems a distant hope, at least in the United States. In her study of "why there is no political demand for new American social welfare rights," the sociologist Sandra Levitsky notes: "Even as the economic strains and psychological stresses on families have intensified, the American public has shown little appetite for translating their private family dilemmas into political demands for new social policies. . . . The ideology of family responsibility for care provision is by all accounts the dominant understanding of social welfare provision in the United States."[10]

If these social, cultural, and political realities were to shift, such that the burdens on family caregivers were lessened and the support available to them were improved, these changes might make a great difference. They still would not, however, fully answer the question of where to find the supportive network that will provide care for older adults with dementia and sustain them in personhood. Recent estimates suggest that 40 percent of all older adults with dementia in the United States live alone, and many have few family members available. The Alzheimer's Association estimates that in 2010 there were 7.2 potential family caregivers (i.e., individuals belonging to kinship categories likely to be called upon and to serve as informal caregivers) for each person over the age of eighty in the United States; this ratio is projected to fall to 4 by 2030 and to 3 by 2050.[11] Leaving aside for a moment the many other reasons that people may not step forward to serve as caregivers for elderly relatives with dementia, these demographic trends mean that even when family members do provide care, such arrangements may be increasingly fragile. If a spouse who is primary caregiver dies, for example, whether adult children or others are available to step in may determine whether an older adult with dementia is left alone and without care, with all the attendant consequences.

Studies of informal family caregivers sometimes embrace an expansive understanding of "family" that includes nonkin who assume kinlike roles and relationships. For example, a recent report on "Families Caring for an Aging America" notes that "the term 'family caregiver' should be used to reflect the diverse nature of older adults' family and helping relationships. Some family caregivers do not have a family kinship or legally defined relationship with the care recipient, but are instead partners, neighbors, or friends."[12] This usage resonates with the use of "fictive kin" terms by some older adults themselves as part of the process by which they create caregiving relations with nonkin.[13] Such terminological imprecision, however, obscures legal and other obstacles that nonkin caregivers may face, and it does not advance efforts to document and understand the complexities of the informal care sector.[14] Some informal caregivers are only ambiguously positioned as "family" relative to the older adult for whom they provide care, such as ex-wives, and studies consistently document that a significant minority are in fact not family members at all, but rather neighbors, friends, and other unrelated persons.[15] Friends who serve as caregivers face obstacles that are important to recognize; they generally do not have power of attorney privileges, are not privy to medical information, and cannot make healthcare decisions, which may limit their ability to provide care.[16]

The sociologist Elena Portacolone, in a recent article about "the precarity of older adults living alone with cognitive impairment," notes: "Informal caregivers, such as family members or adult children, are the people usually nominated as critical providers of care for persons with dementia. Yet they may be emotionally or physically distant or unavailable to older solo dwellers with cognitive impairment."[17]

Unfortunately, we have little empirical information about what happens to older adults with dementia who lack family caregivers. Portacolone's ethnographic research among older adults living alone with cognitive impairment is terribly important. Understandably, given her methods, her research involves a relatively small number of people and focuses on those whose dementia is still in relatively early stages. Older adults with dementia who have neither family nor other nonkin connections available to help meet increasing needs for care and assistance as their capacities recede are "among the most vulnerable in the community and are often alone and estranged from family, neglected and abused, and at risk of receiving inappropriate medical treatment."[18]

This situation is not rare. In the United States, estimates suggest that 16 percent of elderly patients in intensive care units, up to 30 percent of institutionalized elders, and a large but unknown number of others dwelling in the community are "incapacitated and alone."[19] And in contemporary Japan, as Anne Allison's harrowing recent study documents, a combination of political, economic, and cultural shifts have left many older adults adrift and bereft of care, resulting in lonely deaths, unmarked and unmourned, surfacing in stories that haunt the public imagination. Who, Allison asks, "is responsible for caregiving in an era when the family, (once) assigned this responsibility, is losing its capacity to carry it out?"[20] And who, we might further ask, is responsible for sustaining personhood?

Dementia and Friendship

Seeking to document how the relationality of personhood in dementia is enacted beyond the family, I have recently conducted interview-based research with people who have found themselves facing the onset of dementia in a friend. I have also interviewed some family members of people with dementia, and some healthcare professionals who work with them, about their observations and perspectives on the presence or absence of friends in the lives of older adults with dementia. Friendship seems an important topic to explore, if only to counter the assumption that only family members can, will, do, or should remain engaged with older adults who have dementia. The basic idea behind this research is that there may be lessons to learn from those who have found both reasons and ways to maintain relations of friendship after the onset of symptoms that could be shared with others who find themselves confronting similar situations.[21] This research has revealed several ways in which some people who are not bound by family ties refuse and resist inadequate, excessively individualistic visions of the aging person in society and enact an understanding of personhood as relational. Let me just briefly touch on four of these.

First, for some people I have spoken with, the onset of dementia in a friend calls into play an understanding of their *own* personhood as relational. The philosopher Charles Taylor succinctly makes this point: "One cannot be a self on one's own."[22] In this perspective, the onset of dementia in a friend does not erase the relationship but presents difficulties through which one defines oneself, as a friend and a moral self. As the anthropologist Cheryl Mattingly has argued, devastating and unforeseen events present people with moral challenges. Mattingly calls such situations "moral laboratories" to highlight the way that people striving to do the right thing, in circumstances in which it often is unclear, become "researchers and experimenters of their own lives," experimenting with different ways to sustain the moral values, selves, and relationships that they hold most dear. In the process, bad luck can open paths toward developing or revealing unsuspected dimensions of familiar people and relationships: "New projects of becoming may be set in motion through the accidents of fortune. So, a chain of events ... conspire to provide radically altered circumstances and set a new story in motion. Such events ... demand virtues not needed before. Accidents create new situations that demand new or more well-developed virtues in order to even perceive a 'best good' in uncharted waters."[23]

Second, people who have remained engaged as friends after the onset of symptoms also describe dementia as an impetus for personal and interpersonal *transformations* that can involve learning, growth, and unexpected gifts—in addition to sadness and loss. Responding to the new challenges that dementia presents can reveal new sides of oneself, or of other people, and new aspects of relationships. People speak of discovering pleasurably childlike aspects of a friend with dementia, appreciating the new playfulness and physicality that become part of their friendships, and being moved by witnessing the tenderness, thoughtfulness, and devotion that other people show toward the impaired individual. In their accounts, the onset of dementia in a friend appears "tragic," not in the superficial sense of being "sad" or "bad," but in the deeper, richer sense of the tradition of thought associated with tragedy as a classical genre. For indeed, if tragedy holds any lesson at all for its viewers, it is not how to *avoid* tragic outcomes but how to *endure* them, as we observe the nobility with which the protagonist faces his demise, and learn what it means to exhibit virtue in the face of a tragic reversal of fortune.[24]

Third, through experience, people gain specific forms of *knowledge about how to interact well* with the person who has dementia. For example, one may learn what sorts of situations and activities are likely to cause distress, or ways of engaging someone in conversation when their grasp on language has slipped. How the condition affects people can vary enormously, and there is no instruction manual for interacting well with those who have dementia. Still, through experience, friends and family may develop a repertoire of techniques and approaches and a sense of how and when to use them—they develop what we might, if these were medical professionals, call *clinical* knowledge, though we have no special name for it when it is the possession of ordinary laypeople. Like clinical knowledge, it can also be shared and taught, and some people I have interviewed explain that they make a conscious point to teach and to model such knowledge for other people. In so doing, they seek to transform their social world into one more capable of sustaining the personhood of the friend with dementia.

Finally, fourth, a finding that I mention last, even though it often comes first, is that talking about dementia—in other words, making this sometimes difficult and uncomfortable topic "speakable"—can be a critical first step toward approaching it *collectively*, as something for a community to deal with instead of only as an individual problem. Talk does not necessarily accomplish this, of course. Dementia may be (and arguably is) talked about constantly, but so long as such talk frames the problem always as a private matter with which family members struggle, it will have little transformative effect. Yet if the potential exists for social groupings other than or beyond the family to take up the question of dementia and how best to support people living with it, realizing this potential does require that at some point it be named openly as a matter of shared conversation and concern.

Where Friendship Abuts Abandonment

What I had in mind when I embarked on the project of researching friendship with those who have dementia, was a particular kind of situation: a relationship that has already been in place for some time when one of the friends begins to show symptoms of dementia. And many stories that I heard are indeed of that type. But I have also heard stories of situations in which friendships that had begun as more tangential connections became a crucial bulwark against abandonment for persons with dementia who had no family on whom they could rely.

One of the women I interviewed, Glennis, described to me how she helps care for an elderly woman named Jacqueline, originally from China, who never married or had children and now struggles with worsening dementia. Glennis was an administrator at the hospital where Jacqueline used to work as a lab technician and knew her only slightly, but she has become one of several acquaintances working together to help Jacqueline. Together they organized Jacqueline's finances, found an attorney, and paid him to set up the paperwork that needed to be in order. They also arranged for a caregiver to come every day to the apartment where Jacqueline lives alone to help her clean up, make her lunch, and give her medications. One had taken primary charge of Jacqueline's medical appointments, another of her finances, and all arranged to take Jacqueline on social outings. Developing and sustaining these arrangements had been challenging, however, in part because friendships are not as readily legible to the state as kinship relations or business transactions. Glennis recounted that Sally, who manages Jacqueline's finances, had been reported to Adult Protective Services by a bank teller who became suspicious of her and had been investigated; and she was very hurt and upset by the experience and had wanted to step away from the whole arrangement.

Sarah, a professional woman in her early 60s in Seattle, having heard about my research from a mutual friend, sought me out to tell me about her involvement with her neighbor Gloria, who lived alone in her single-family home and had developed dementia. For nearly fifteen years, the two had been in the habit of meeting early each morning to walk their dogs together around the neighborhood. Over the years, as Gloria had become progressively more impaired, they had sustained this routine, and it had become ever more important—as a social connection that persisted after many others faded away and as a daily check on Gloria's well-being. Rachel was in touch with Gloria's long-term boyfriend (who remained a loyal presence but lived in his own house a half-hour drive away) as well as her sister (who lived out of state), and she would call to alert them if she saw or learned of anything worrisome concerning Gloria, her dog, or her house.

Sometimes it was family members seeking to step up as caregivers who became aware that seemingly random people had taken on what they regarded as an outsized role in the daily life of the person with dementia. Joan, a woman in her 50s, saw her mother's attachment to staff at her neighborhood Costco as a symptom of her dementia, which had already affected her ability to keep up relations with friends of long standing:

> I'd been noticing . . . her details just—they weren't connecting. But at that point already her friendships had slipped from being true friends to going to Costco and interacting with the people who work in the aisles. Those were her new "friends" because there was little—you didn't have to put much energy into it. You came and saw them. They were busy doing other things. But she went to Costco all the time because those were her *friends*. Of course, she can't go to Costco without buying stuff, so then her house starts filling up with paper products. . . . I tell you, I didn't buy paper products for a *year* after I moved her out. I don't need paper towels. I don't need toilet paper! I saw her basement piled high—because she didn't put it away, she just piled it up. So, those were the things I was seeing. And, um, I truly thought she had all these friends but then I realized they were just friendly cashiers. . . . I've

been to Costco with her, and it was frustrating to me because she is—unfiltered. She's the person on the elevator who talks to everyone standing there, whether you really want to hear it or not. So, my observation was that these people were polite and kind and busy. But . . . they weren't very deep friendships.

I actually met Glennis, Sarah, and Joan in person, and I was able to sit down and talk with each of them and ask questions, but there are many more such stories that I have not been able to follow up on in the same way. For example, a geriatric social worker, Tina, described to me one of the "strange relationships" she had witnessed over the years she had worked in this field:

I've had strange relationships over the years, people that have picked up these people in their lives like grocery store clerks. Yeah. Sometimes just very tangential. They've ended up being their power of attorney because the person had no one else, and they ended up like bringing them groceries every other day and helping them, and giving them rides, and sort of becoming friends, and they just had this rather cursory relationship to begin with. Odd how it happens. But well, the woman would go to that grocery store just about every day. And so over the years he just recognized her and was having small chats with her, and then having longer chats with her; and then one day, he just said, "Can I *bring* you your groceries?" . . . And so that kind of shifted the relationship, and [he] brought her home and started realizing those common needs. Some support. Yep. And when I actually did the [durable power of attorney] document with her she was crystal clear that she trusted this guy.

Such trust is not always well deserved, of course. The bank teller who, as Glennis recounted, called Adult Protective Services to report a concern that Sally might be exploiting Jacqueline, was doubtless acting conscientiously, even if mistakenly in this case; the teller knew that older adults with dementia who are alone may be vulnerable to exploitation or abuse at the hands of unscrupulous strangers who become their "new friends." But it is also true, even if less readily acknowledged, that vulnerable elders may be abused or exploited by family members as well. And with tangential friendships as with family members, relationships can be complex, with seemingly incompatible elements of exploitation and care. Consider, for example, Tina's account of another "strange relationship":

> The patient has since passed away, and probably the caregiver too. She was 104 the last time I talked to her; the patient was 84, she's 20 years older. Met him in a gas station. A strange relationship. But she ended up . . . [*laughs*] . . . becoming his power of attorney, letting him live in her house, doing all of his laundry and cooking and cleaning and all of that, 20 years older than he was. He died when she was 104, and she was still ambulatory and cognitively intact and amazing. Might be still alive, for all I know. She was stubborn. But she actually ended up exploiting him. . . . I saw him very regularly, because he had nobody; she didn't really start stepping up until probably about five years before he died. And ended up robbing him of his entire life's savings, which wasn't much. And he knew she was taking his money; and she would ask him for money and he would give it to her. And when it was reported, he kept saying, "No, I wanted her to have it. I wanted her to have it." But [from] the things that he had told *me*, previous to that happening, I knew what he was planning to use that money for and why he had saved it for all those years. And it wasn't very much money, but it was all he had, and he ended up on Medicaid and in an adult family home. . . . But she was interesting, because in some ways she really was his friend. She took him to church, she socialized with him, she fed him, she knew him probably better than anybody else. He would have considered her his best friend, without a doubt, and the exploitation came along later. It was a crime of opportunity for her, and probably partially because of her son who was a drug addict and violent, and he probably was strong arming her as well. But she was an interesting lady. And the fact that she met this guy at a gas station and then somehow stayed in contact with him and . . . . It was odd. It's just so interesting how that happens.

Methodologically, this friendship research itself has been a bit "odd" in that it is defined by a focus on people who have in common a particular kind of situation that they occupy—each is self-identified as the friend of someone who is living with dementia. As such, these individuals occupy a shared moral space of commitment and care, and they share a felt delegation or categorization as part of a community that includes the person with dementia. They do not, however, share geographic location, occupation, or membership in any particular social or cultural group. Recruitment has therefore been an interesting challenge; how is one to find such people? I have pursued a variety of approaches: I have placed flyers in doctors' offices and senior centers and posted notices on Facebook, Craigslist, and Nextdoor. But in fact, most of the people I have interviewed have come to me through introductions provided by people I know: colleagues, students, neighbors, women I work out with at my gym, friends of mine. As I mentioned a bit earlier, the importance of talk about dementia among friends has emerged as one of the *findings* from this research — but quite to my surprise, talk about dementia among friends has also turned out to be a vital *method* allowing the research to happen. Whether fortunately or unfortunately, it seems that nearly everyone I talk to knows of someone who is taking care of an unrelated older adult with dementia, and I become aware of many more such situations, if only in a glancing, indirect, out-of-the-corner-of-the-eye manner.

A few examples:

- Jeremy, another geriatric social worker whom I interviewed, told me about a client who had asked him to help her find out how her former neighbor was doing. He was an elderly man with dementia who had lived alone in an apartment near hers, in a low-income housing development. When the building was razed and rebuilt as part of an urban redevelopment scheme, the two neighbors were relocated to different buildings in parts of the city quite distant from each other. She was unable to visit him and was worried about how he was managing without her help.
- A colleague at my university, with whom I was chatting about my research, told me that the mail carrier in her neighborhood regularly delivers meals to a particular old woman on the route who lives alone and is impaired.[25]
- I met for coffee with a law professor in Seattle whom I had contacted to ask about her research in the field of elder law. When I told her about my interest in dementia and friendship, she told me about someone in her neighborhood who has taken on the care of the elderly woman next door, who lives alone and has dementia.

- A real estate professional named Ben, with whom I met for reasons having nothing to do with work, turned out to be a very friendly, chatty person. He asked me about my job, and I briefly described my research. He volunteered a story about his aunt and uncle, who, when he was growing up, lived on a large piece of land on Whidbey Island (north of Seattle). They had, he told me, taken in a man from the town who had no family and who had developed dementia. The aunt and uncle had let this man, whose name was Bobby, live in a trailer on their property, and they took care of him. Ben recalled, as a teenager, being asked to come spend afternoons and evenings looking after him—he referred to it, with a laugh, as "Bobbysitting."

What should one do with such stories? Their ubiquity suggests, at least, that stories like this stand out in people's minds—they are memorable. At the same time, these stories seem to be shared and told *only* when I come asking about them, in line with my peculiar interests. Are such stories memorable because they are so *unusual*? Or are they perhaps very *common*? Absent reliable information, it is difficult to know. We can read these stories as frightening glimpses of a looming abyss of social abandonment, the full dimensions of which we may never even know— or we can read them as heartening evidence of the capacity of ordinary people to see and respond to the needs of fellow human beings in what David Graeber calls "the communism of everyday social relations."[26]

Toward Relational Citizenship

The idea of relational personhood, by presenting us with the question of *which* network of relationships will enact it for older adults with dementia, has led us to consider first families, then friendships, and finally the "strange relationships" that may arise where friendship abuts abandonment. About these latter, it is perhaps worth noting how many of them concern interactions taking place in the public sphere of commerce. The grocery store clerk who became deeply involved in caring for one isolated elderly woman with dementia, the Costco staff who figured as "friends" for another, the very old woman who became the best friend and live-in caregiver (and eventual exploiter) of a man with dementia whom she had met at a gas station—all of these examples point toward the marketplace as a potentially important site of social connections and care poised in between the family and the state. Interestingly, the philosopher Hilde Lindemann specifically calls out interactions with grocery store clerks as among the occasions in which the social practice of personhood—or, as she calls it, "holding someone in personhood"—happens:

> You're leaving the convenience store and an entering stranger smiles at you and says it's getting colder outside; he's holding you in personhood. Or the clerk doesn't even glance at you when she takes your money; she's letting you go. As one-time events, these exchanges neither make nor mar you, but if no clerk ever looked at you . . . the many little instances you might experience of being let go could make it very difficult to hold yourself in personhood.[27]

In each of the domains we have considered, we find people who make great efforts, working with great creativity and care, to sustain others whose very lives as well as their personhood dementia has rendered precarious. Yet each of these domains has limits, and none of these situations or kinds of relationships can be reliably counted on to come together as and when needed. Family may rally and come to the support of older adults with dementia—but not all have family, and not all family members can or will rise to the occasion. Friends and neighbors and acquaintances may see and respond to the needs of an older adult who is impaired and alone, as Glennis and others have done—but such arrangements may be fragile, and temporary, or they may not coalesce at all. Grocery store clerks and others who encounter them in the public sphere of commerce may respond to older adults with dementia in ways that exceed their job descriptions or the ordinary expectations of transactional interactions—but most probably will not. Luck, chance, and caprice play a large role, and the specter of abandonment remains haunting. The question of who will respond to older adults with dementia thus also leads us directly into questions about the purpose of the state and the meaning of citizenship. Can and should the state step in where family and civil society fail?

If citizenship is understood as a property possessed by autonomous individuals, people with dementia who are unable to perform autonomy and independence cannot be citizens and must be spoken for by others. The mechanisms through which that can happen, at least in the United States, are few and rather dire: state agencies such as Adult Protective Services and various forms of legal guardianship, each of which involves taking away a person's civil rights.[28]

When an elderly person with dementia ends up, for example, in a hospital emergency room *without* having formally designated a person to act as a healthcare proxy, and a major medical decision must be made, practitioners try to identify and contact a legally authorized surrogate decision-maker. Laws in each state, called "default surrogate consent statutes," specify the priority order of individuals who can in such circumstances be appointed as surrogate decision-makers.[29] These statutes vary, and the list of eligible categories can be longer or shorter. In twenty-three states and Washington DC, "close friend" does appear on this list, always as a last priority. In Washington state, where I lived for twenty years, the list of authorized categories is very short and does not include "friend" or even very many categories of "family": (1) spouse or registered domestic partner; (2) adult children; (3) parents; and (4) adult siblings. This means that even if there is a cousin, niece or nephew, former sister-in-law, neighbor, or friend who has been very involved in helping a person out with daily needs, unless that person has already been formally appointed as power of attorney, he or she cannot legally make medical decisions in this situation without a court order.

When an elderly person with dementia has no legal guardian and no one who satisfies the default consent statutes, a physician may contact Adult Protective Services, and they may, in turn, petition the court to appoint a guardian. If the judge agrees, she or he will appoint a guardian ad litem, who is paid by the court and whose job is to investigate this particular case and make a recommendation as to the best course of action. If no family can be identified who are judged suitable, the guardian ad litem may recommend that a professional guardian be appointed. The costs of these services are paid by the estate of the ward to whom they are assigned. As a result of this built-in conflict of interest, such guardianship arrangements, which are supposed to protect vulnerable older adults from abuse, can themselves create conditions ripe for abuse and exploitation, as vividly depicted in a recent journalistic account of the predatory practices of some unscrupulous professional guardians.[30] Older adults who are poor have no estates to draw upon, and few professional guardians will agree to work with them. In such cases, the court must wait until a volunteer guardian is available (these volunteers are often lawyers, judges, or others involved in the field of eldercare, who take on this work on a pro bono basis). A director of home healthcare services in Seattle, who in the course of her work encounters many "unbefriended" older adults with dementia, estimated that the whole process of getting a guardian appointed generally takes about a year.

Recognizing that people with dementia and other impairments are ill served by conceptions of citizenship premised on the need to perform autonomy, some have sought to rethink the concept of citizenship in a relational mode. As Rachel Adams notes, the image of the citizen as an autonomous individual remains implicit not only in social contract theories but even in disability rights discourses. She notes that, according to the United Nations Convention on the Rights of Persons with Disabilities (UNCRPD),

> Even the most severely disabled persons should be entitled, to the best of their capacities, to make decisions about their own care. Given the isolation and voicelessness of people with disabilities throughout much of human history, the collective demand for self-determination represented a radical step forward. But more recently, critics have observed that the emphasis on independence and productivity within the mainstream disability rights movement excludes those who are unable to represent themselves.[31]

Adams cites the philosopher Martha Nussbaum, who has sought to develop a version of Rawlsian social contract theory revised to place human interdependency at its center: "In the design of the political conception of the person out of which basic political principles grow, we build in an acknowledgment that we are needy temporal animal beings who begin as babies and end, often, in other forms of dependency. We draw attention to these areas of vulnerability, insisting that rationality and sociability are themselves temporal, having growth, maturity, and (if time permits) decline."[32]

Central to Nussbaum's account is a statement of key human "capabilities" that she argues are necessary for human flourishing, and therefore to her "noncontractarian account of care":

Although my view insists that human beings are inevitably dependent and interdependent, and holds that dignity may be found in relations of dependency, citizens enjoy full equality only when they are capable of exercising the whole range of capabilities. At times this may have to be done through a guardian . . . but the goal is always to put the person herself in the position of full capability . . . not because of social productivity, but because it is humanly good.[33]

In other words, in place of the image of the autonomous rational individual upon which social contract theory conceptions of citizenship have been premised, Nussbaum proposes a new and arguably less inadequate depiction of the person. She proposes envisioning the individual as a needy, embodied, temporal, interdependent being and contends that beginning from this better starting point will allow for the development of a new and more just understanding of citizenship as relational.

The political philosopher and ethnographer of medicine Jeannette Pols, meanwhile, has recently articulated a different conception of "relational citizenship" that, instead of positing a new-and-improved definition of "the citizen as a particular individual," explores citizenship as "a matter of sociality."[34] In so doing, this approach "moves citizenship away from the relationship between individual and state toward the relationship between citizens."[35] It also opens up the possibility that there may in fact be *multiple* different ways of enacting relations of citizenship, creatively devised in response to the specificities of their particular situations, by people in different social locations. The task, then, is not to select or invent the one, true, best image of the citizen upon which to build one's theory, but rather to build an expanded repertoire of ways of enacting relations that support inclusion and participation. By carefully documenting and analyzing these, ethnographic research can, in this view, expand and enrich not only understandings but potentially also practices of citizenship. As Pols writes,

This notion of citizenship is a tool for studying social relationships empirically, to find out what works and why, to what type of social spaces these relationships lead, and what materials and values keep these social spaces together. It allows for an analysis of how the parties renegotiate norms rather than assume that . . . people with intellectual disabilities will adapt to existing norms. Differences are considered part of interactions, and hence the way participants find ways to deal with differences can be studied as possibilities for organizing relationships elsewhere.[36]

Here, then, our exploration into seemingly hopeless endings leads to a somewhat hopeful conclusion. To return to our original questions: What happens to older adults with dementia who are without family, and in some cases without even friends—and how might the problems for them reflect "a deficient conception of the person in society"? The simplest and truest answer is that we know far too little about what happens in such situations; not nearly enough attention has been paid. The slightly less cryptic answer is that what happens to such people can really vary: How they are, or are not, recognized and embraced and supported by others matters enormously for how they live, whether and how they suffer, and how they die. The somewhat hopeful aspect of all this is that all around us, quietly and with little fanfare, and sometimes against great odds, there can be found ordinary people who respond to impaired older adults with compassion, care, and creativity. It is perhaps to be expected that this will happen in homes and clinics and care institutions—but we can take heart at finding that it also happens in more surprising ways and places. In neighborhoods and grocery stores, in workplaces and gas stations, on postal routes, and in conversations among friends, people can and sometimes do engage with impaired and isolated older adults in ways that sustain them within a social embrace and enact relational personhood and citizenship. Ethnographic research has something positive to contribute by documenting these creative interventions and holding them up for all of us to consider, admire, reflect upon, and learn from. We have much to learn, and much to do; for me, and for each of us, evening is falling quickly.

Notes

I gratefully acknowledge receipt in 2014–2015 of support for research on dementia and friendship from the Fetzer Institute, a private philanthropic foundation whose mission is to "inspire and serve a global movement grounded in connection that transforms the world into a more loving home for all" (see www.fetzer.org).

This research is discussed in greater detail in two works by Janelle S. Taylor cited in endnote 21. I am deeply grateful to the individuals who have shared their experiences and reflections with me, to the editors of this volume for their editorial guidance and leadership, and to the many friends, colleagues, and students who have provided indispensable advice and comments along the way. Special thanks to Sharon Kaufman, Sarah Lamb, Caitrin Lynch, Priti Ramamurthy, China Scherz, and Lynn Thomas.

1. W. Ladson Hinton and Sue Levkoff, "Constructing Alzheimer's: Narratives of Lost Identities, Confusion, and Loneliness in Old Age," *Culture, Medicine and Psychiatry* 23, no. 4 (December 1999): 453–75, 461.

2. Janelle S. Taylor, "On Recognition, Caring, and Dementia," *Medical Anthropology Quarterly* 22, no. 4 (December 2008): 313–35, 326.

3. Cynthia M. Boyd, Jonathan Darer, Chad Boult, Linda P. Fried, Lisa Boult, and Albert W. Wu, "Clinical Practice Guidelines and Quality of Care for Older Patients with Multiple Comorbid Diseases: Implications for Pay for Performance," *Journal of the American Medical Association* 294, no. 6 (August 2005): 716–24; Lauren E. Griffith, Andrea Gruneir, Kathryn Fisher, Dilzayn Panjwani, Sima Gandhi, Li Sheng, Amiram Gafni, Christopher Patterson, Maureen Markle-Reid, and Jenny Ploeg, "Patterns of Health Service Use in Community Living Older Adults with Dementia and Comorbid Conditions: A Population-Based Retrospective Cohort Study in Ontario, Canada," *BioMed Central Geriatrics* 16, no. 1 (October 2016): 177–87; Mary E. Tinetti, Terri R. Fried, and Cynthia M. Boyd, "Designing Health Care for the Most Common Chronic Condition— Multimorbidity," *Journal of the American Medical Association* 307, no. 23 (June 2012): 2493–94.

4. Jennifer L. Wolff and Brenda Spillman, "Older Adults Receiving Assistance with Physician Visits and Prescribed Medications and their Family Caregivers: Prevalence, Characteristics, and Hours of Care," *Journals of Gerontology, Series B: Psychological Sciences and Social Sciences* 69, no. 7 (November 2014): S65–S72.

5. Carol Levine, *Always on Call: When Illness Turns Families into Caregivers*, 2nd ed. (Nashville: Vanderbilt University Press, 2004); Cheryl Mattingly, Lone Grøn, and Lotte Meinert, "Chronic Homework in Emerging Borderlands of Healthcare," *Culture, Medicine and Psychiatry* 35, no. 3 (September 2011): 347–75.

6. Joan M. Teno, Pedro L. Gozalo, Julie Bynum, Natalie Leland, Susan C. Miller, Nancy E. Morden, Thomas Scupp, David C. Goodman, and Vincent Mor, "Change in End-of-Life Care for Medicare Beneficiaries: Site of Death, Place of Care, and Health Care Transitions in 2000, 2005, and 2009," *Journal of the American Medical Association* 309, no. 5 (February 2013): 470–77.

7. Ann Bookman and Mona Harrington, "Family Caregivers: A Shadow Workforce in the Geriatric Healthcare System?," *Journal of Health Politics, Policy, and Law* 32, no. 6 (December 2007): 1005–41; Susan C. Reinhard, Carol Levine, and Sarah Samis, *Home Alone: Family Caregivers Providing Complex Medical Care* (Washington, DC: AARP/United Hospital Fund, 2012).

8. Joseph E. Gaugler, Robert L. Kane, Rosalie A. Kane, and Robert Newcomer, "Unmet Care Needs and Key Outcomes in Dementia," *Journal of the American Geriatrics Society* 53, no. 12 (December 2005): 2098–105; Vicki A. Freedman, and Brenda C. Spillman, "Disability and Care Needs among Older Americans," *Milbank Quarterly* 92, no. 3 (September 2014): 509–41.

9. National Academies of Sciences, Engineering, and Medicine, *Families Caring for an Aging America* (Washington, DC: National Academies Press, 2016), 256.

10. Sandra R. Levitsky, *Caring for Our Own: Why There Is No Political Demand for New American Social Welfare Rights* (Oxford: Oxford University Press, 2015), 4.

11. Alzheimer's Association, "2016 Alzheimer's Diseases Facts & Figures," *Alzheimer's & Dementia* 12, no. 4 (April 2016): 459–509.

12. National Academies of Sciences, Engineering, and Medicine, *Families Caring for An Aging America*, 20.

13. "Fictive kin" is described in Margaret K. Nelson's "Fictive Kin, Families We Choose, and Voluntary Kin: What Does the Discourse Tell Us?," *Journal of Family Theory & Review* 5, no. 4 (December 2013): 259–81. The process of creating caregiving relationships with nonkin is explained in Marieke Voorpostel, "Just Like Family: Fictive Kin Relationships in the Netherlands," *Journals of Gerontology, Series B: Psychological Sciences and Social Sciences* 68, no. 5 (September 2013): 816–24.

14. For more on the obstacles faced by nonkin caregivers, see Anna Muraco and Karen Frederiksen-Goldsen, "'That's What Friends Do': Informal Caregiving for Chronically Ill Midlife and Older Lesbian, Gay, and Bisexual Adults," *Journal of Social and Personal Relationships* 28, no. 8 (December 2011): 1078–93; Catherine M. Burns, Amy P. Abernethy, Eleanora Dal Grande, and David C. Currow, "Uncovering an Invisible Network of Direct Caregivers at the End of Life: A Population Study," *Palliative Medicine* 27, no. 7 (July 2013): 608–15. For more on the complexities of informal care, see Tracy A. Lapierre and Nora Keating, "Characteristics and Contributions of Non-Kin Carers of Older Adults: A Closer Look at Friends and Neighbours," *Ageing and Society* 33 no. 8 (November 2013): 1442–68, 1443.

15. For more on the ambiguous positions of informal caregivers who are ex-wives, see Teresa M. Cooney, Christine Proulx, Linley A. Snyder-Rivas, and Jac-

quelyn Benson, "Role Ambiguity among Women Providing Care for Ex-Husbands," *Journal of Women & Aging* 26, no. 1 (January 2014): 84–104. For more on unrelated persons as caregivers, see Judith C. Barker, "Neighbors, Friends, and Other Nonkin Caregivers of Community-Living Dependent Elders," *Journals of Gerontology Series B: Psychological Sciences and Social Sciences* 57, no. 3 (May 2002): S158–67; Andrew Nocon and Maggie Pearson, "The Roles of Friends and Neighbors in Providing Support for Older People," *Ageing & Society* 20, no. 3 (May 2000): 341–67; Lapierre and Keating, "Characteristics and Contributions of Non-Kin Carers of Older People"; Catherine M. Burns, Amy P. Abernethy, Eleanora Dal Grande, and David C. Currow, "Uncovering an Invisible Network of Direct Caregivers at the End of Life: A Population Study," *Palliative Medicine* 27, no. 7 (July 2013): 608–15.

16. Anna Muraco and Karen Frederiksen-Goldsen, "'That's What Friends Do': Informal Caregiving for Chronically Ill Midlife and Older Lesbian, Gay, and Bisexual Adults," *Journal of Social and Personal Relationships* 28, no. 8 (December 2011): 1078–93.

17. Elena Portacolone, Robert L. Rubinstein, Kenneth E. Covinsky, Jodi Halpern, and Julene K. Johnson, "The Precarity of Older Adults Living Alone with Cognitive Impairment," *Gerontologist* 59, no. 2 (March 2019): 271–80.

18. Robin Bandy, Greg A. Sachs, Kianna Montz, Lev Inger, Robert W. Bandy, and Alexia M. Torke, "Wishard Volunteer Advocates Program: An Intervention for At-Risk, Incapacitated, Unbefriended Adults," *Journal of the American Geriatrics Society* 62, no. 11 (November 2014): 2171–79.

19. Naomi Karp and Erica Wood, *Incapacitated and Alone: Health Care Decision-Making for the Unbefriended Elderly* (American Bar Association Commission on Law and Aging, July 2003); Timothy W. Farrell, Eric Widera, Lisa Rosenberg, Craig D. Rubin, Aanand D. Naik, Ursula Braun, Alexia Torke, Ina Li, Caroline Vitale, and Joseph Shega, Ethics, Clinical Practice and Models of Care, and Public Policy Committees of the American Geriatrics Society, "AGS Position Statement: Making Medical Treatment Decisions for Unbefriended Older Adults," *Journal of the American Geriatrics Society* 65, no. 1 (January 2017): 14–15.

20. Anne Allison, *Precarious Japan* (Durham: Duke University Press, 2013), 159.

21. Janelle S. Taylor, "Should Old Acquaintance Be Forgot?: Friendship in the Face of Dementia," in *Successful Aging as a Contemporary Obsession: Global Perspectives*, ed. Sarah Lamb (New Brunswick, NJ: Rutgers University Press, 2017), 126–38, and Janelle S. Taylor, "Engaging with Dementia: Moral Experiments in Art and Friendship," *Culture, Medicine and Psychiatry* 41, no. 2 (April 2017): 284–303.

22. Charles Taylor, *Sources of the Self* (Cambridge, MA: Harvard University Press, 1989), 34, quoted in Cheryl Mattingly, *Moral Laboratories: Family Peril and the Struggle for a Good Life* (Berkeley, CA: University of California Press, 2014), 22.

23. Mattingly, *Moral Laboratories*, 82.

24. Janelle S. Taylor, "The Story Catches You and You Fall Down: Tragedy, Ethnography, and 'Cultural Competence,'" *Medical Anthropology Quarterly* 17, no. 2 (June 2003): 159–81, 163.

25. See also Zoey Poll, "In France, Elder Care Comes with the Mail," New Yorker, October 9, 2019.

26. David Graeber, *Debt: The First 5,000 Years* (New York: Melville House, 2011), 95.

27. Hilde Lindemann, *Holding and Letting Go: The Social Practice of Personal Identities* (Oxford: Oxford University Press, 2014), 203.

28. Martha E. Leatherman, and Katherine E. Goethe, "Substituted Decision Making: Elder Guardianship," *Journal of Psychiatric Practice* 15, no. 6 (November 2009): 470–76, and Pamela Teaster, "The Wards of Public Guardians: Voices of the Unbefriended," *Family Relations* 51, no. 4 (October 2002): 344–50.

29. American Bar Association Commission on Law and Aging, "Default Surrogate Consent Statutes," 2018, https://www.americanbar.org/content/dam/aba/administrative/law_aging/2014_default_surrogate_consent_statutes.authcheckdam.pdf, and Erin S. DeMartino, David M. Dudzinksi, and Daniel B. Kramer, "Who Decides When a Patient Can't?: Statutes on Alternate Decision Makers," *New England Journal of Medicine* 376, no. 15 (April 2017): 1478–82.

30. Rachel Aviv, "How the Elderly Lose Their Rights," *New Yorker*, October 2, 2017, https://www.newyorker.com/magazine/2017/10/09/how-the-elderly-lose-their-rights.

31. Rachel Adams, "Disability Life Writing and the Problem of Dependency in the Autobiography of Gaby Brimmer," *Journal of Medical Humanities* 38, no. 1 (March 2017): 39–50, 41.

32. Martha Nussbaum, *Frontiers of Justice: Disability, Nationality, Species Membership* (Cambridge, MA: Harvard University Press, 2006), 160.

33. Ibid., 218.

34. Jeannette Pols, "Analyzing Social Spaces: Relational Citizenship for Patients Leaving Mental Health Care Institutions," *Medical Anthropology* 35, no. 2 (March–April 2016): 177–92, 177.

35. Ibid., 188.

36. Ibid.

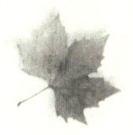

CHAPTER NINE

The Priority of Social and Physical Function
Older Adults in the CAPABLE Program

SARAH L. SZANTON AND

JANIECE TAYLOR

The notion of "successful aging," as noted in previous chapters, puts the onus on the individual adult to have a certain kind of older age. This "success" is unattainable by many due to life course racial discrimination, poverty, genetics, or other reasons. In our work, we focus on optimizing the everyday lives of older adults. More than 90 percent of older adults wish to age in their current homes or neighborhoods.[1] "Aging in place," also called "aging in community," provides a better quality of life for older adults and their families, and it is more cost effective for society. However, there are currently no systems in place to support this goal, unlike other goals supported by the majority of society. For more than a century, for instance, there has been free universal education due to a societal consensus that an educated workforce is better for families, individuals, employers, and the economy. There are disparities in the quality of that education, but it is free and universally provided.

While there is a consensus that it is better for individuals, families, employers (to decrease absenteeism of family members), and the economy for older adults to age at home, there is no system of similar supports. There is not even universal assessment of the ability to age at home. The Medicare Wellness Visit can assess older citizens' ability to perform basic and instrumental activities of daily living (ADLs) such as bathing, grooming, or walking across a small room, all daily tasks essential to providing the self-care that enables one to age in place; however, the Medicare Wellness Visit is underused and is not completed in peoples' homes.[2]

In this chapter, having set the scene for aging in place, we will tie aging in place to community participation and address why it matters. Next we consider health disparities that impact one's ability to participate in the community, as well as the important role of function and self-care to community involvement. We then broaden the frame to introduce the society-to-cells resilience framework that underpins interventions that address a person within a family, community, and society. And we describe a program guided by the resilience framework, the Community Aging in Place, Advancing Better Living for Elders (CAPABLE) program. Finally, we end with a case from the CAPABLE program and identify a number of generalizable lessons for helping older adults age in place.

Why Does Community Participation Matter, and What Hinders It?

Although medical care is a key factor in health, it accounts for only 20 percent of people's health outcomes.[3] The other 80 percent of health is shaped by structural determinants such as housing, transit opportunities, adequate food, and health behaviors.[4] In the medical framework, older adults are viewed as the bodies they have, afflicted by diseases and symptoms. This is a body that will wear out on a more or less predictable schedule based on age and risk factors. Social determinants structure these diseases and symptoms, and they heavily influence access to treatment, quality of life, and health-care costs. In examining what older adults need, it is important to address the whole person, which includes the "non-health" factors that affect health.

One of the elements critical for living a high-quality "seniorhood" is the ability to participate in family and community activities. Unfortunately, there are disparities in every factor affecting participation, from gait speed to heart-failure symptoms to hospitalizations.[5] Community participation enriches the entire community and is possible when older adults can act with ease and without pain. As a society, to harness the wisdom and perspective of all older adults, we need to support their functioning. They place a high priority on function, both with respect to the ability to provide self-care, such as bathing and dressing, and to get around in the community.[6] To be able to garden, to walk a grandchild to the school bus, or to volunteer at a Head Start center are examples of what makes for a quality seniorhood filled with meaning and purpose.

Important contributions from sociology, anthropology, and psychology show that late life can be a time of increased wisdom, perspective, and generativity.[7] Creating the circumstances to build on and express these positive abilities is important not only for the individuals themselves but also for their families, communities, and the societies in which they live. From this more holistic view, it is clear that, as a nation, we should prioritize developing the conditions necessary for the best possible physical and emotional function to support the whole generative person. Physical and emotional function are underrecognized by systems of care but essential to a positive experience as an older adult. Even the simple task of improving how people handle stairs can support the whole generative person and improve her quality of life while aging.

A Theoretical Backdrop to Community Participation and Meaningful Engagement

A theoretical way of looking at resilience is the Society to Cells Resilience Framework.[8] As illustrated in figure 1, this framework posits that society, community, family, and individual factors can promote resilience. Although many resilience theories focus primarily on the individual, examining such

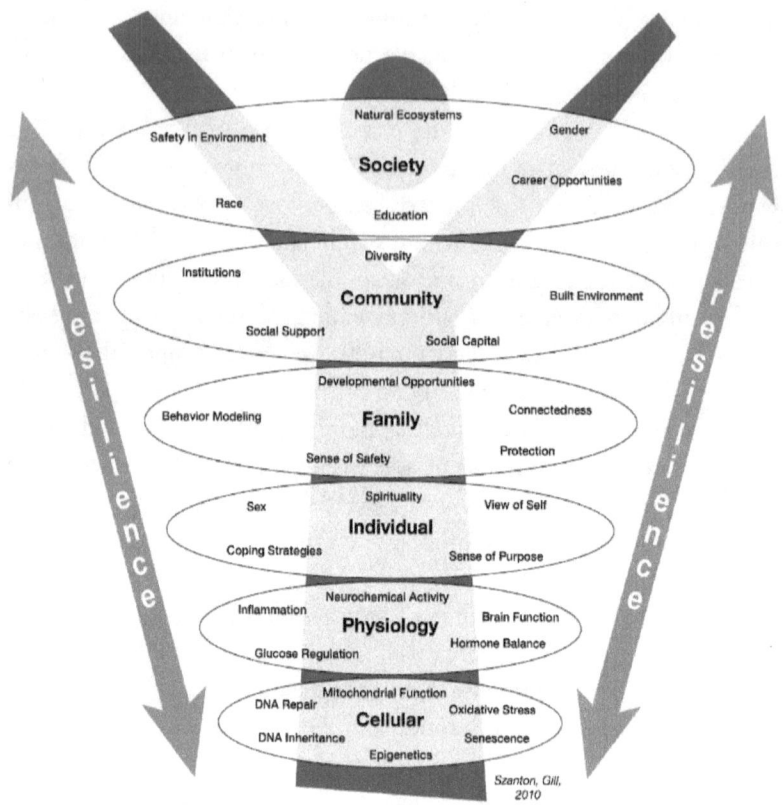

FIGURE 1. Society to Cells Resilience Framework

things as optimism, coping, or spirituality, the Society to Cells Resilience Framework takes into account the simultaneously influencing factors from multiple levels (environment to individual) to yield greater and longer-lasting changes for people. For example, the same arthritis pain and lower leg weakness may occur in two different people with the same biology at birth, but one may have access to a community with more resources or more educational opportunities than the other has, and that person may respond more resiliently than the person with less access to resources, even at the cellular level, because of these differences.

Unique to the resilience framework is the idea that individuals and families can develop increased capacity through a health challenge (such as pain or dialysis) that they can later generalize and apply in other health challenges.[9] This type of resilience in health is called rebound, and it characterizes individuals who have thrived or flourished in spite of or because of challenges, as in post-traumatic growth.[10] An older adult may be able to view the next challenge knowing how he or she has improved with those challenges that have come before. Also, just as there are particularly vulnerable periods in life, the Society to Cells Resilience Framework posits that there are particularly resilient or "plastic" periods in the lives of individuals and families. People in certain phases of life are more likely to develop new habits or take in important information. In our work, we have found, for example, that those providing daily care for a family member with dementia or stroke, although the work is demanding, can find deep strength and connection in the daily care of the family member that they can then carry into other relationships and the development of other skills.[11] One way to leverage this resilience is to focus on preserved abilities, interests, values, and purpose in life.[12]

To put this theoretical resilience base into action with older adults, it is important to shift from provider-centric, disease-specific biomedical approaches to person-centered, community-focused approaches. Unlike patient-centered care, "person-centered" care is concerned with the person over time, not just in visits, and takes the perspective of what the person experiences as health and his or her priorities.[13] In this approach, we build on the assets rather than the deficits of the participating persons, families, and communities. Person-centered approaches take what the older adults want to accomplish in life as the focus and wrap the parts of the intervention around those goals.

One person-centered approach is behavioral activation, which helps people adapt to challenges.[14] In this model, a person sets small, attainable goals, builds a plan to meet those goals, and focuses on how she or he feels in attaining those goals to reinforce the behavioral activation in a positive cycle.[15] Use of behavioral activation to address challenges can not only improve emotional and physical function outcomes but also lead to sustainable behaviors that an older adult can maintain over extended periods of time. It is possible to unlock resilience at any age and stage if a caregiver understands an older adult's own motivation and most important goals and works to alter the environment to achieve these goals.

As an example, we describe the CAPABLE program. This is a multicomponent intervention to reduce disability, ameliorate depressive symptoms, and support activity meaningful to older adults. This person-centered approach includes strategies from multiple levels (from home environment to individual) to promote resilience among members of our target population. The person-centered approach uses the individual participant's interests and abilities, which helps promote resilience.

The CAPABLE program was designed to improve health for older populations and society by addressing both personal and environmental factors that create difficulty in performing activities of daily living (ADLs) such as bathing, dressing, and grooming, as well as instrumental activities of daily living (IADLs) such as managing medications, preparing food, and doing light housekeeping at home. CAPABLE extends ABLE (Advancing Better Living for Elders), which improved participants' quality of life, strengthened their ability to perform ADLs and IADLs, and reduced their fear of falling and risk of mortality through a program involving six sessions conducted by occupational therapists and a physical therapist to help them learn new ways of functioning at home.[16] CAPABLE augments this approach with four sessions conducted by a nurse to address pain management, medications, depressive symptoms, strength, and balance. We hypothesized that addressing common medical challenges with the addition of a nurse would support and intensify improvements in functional ability.[17] CAPABLE also extended environmental modifications to include home repairs through a handyman. In the case of older adults who have lived in their homes a long time and have limited financial resources, there are often holes in their floors, shaky bannisters, or crumbling outdoor stairs. CAPABLE reduces the impact of disability among low-income older adults by addressing both individual capacities and the home environment. Here are comments made by two program participants:

> I felt like a million dollars when I realized I could get to the mailbox, even when winter comes, and not be afraid of falling. (Female, 78 years old)

> I couldn't go up and down the steps. I couldn't comb my hair, I couldn't do my bath, there was a lot of things I couldn't do. Now I can do better.

Oh, I don't want to let them quit. I want to continue with them but if they do they might can't help nobody else, I can understand that. Very, very helpful. (Female, 75 years old)

Both women quoted above were able to rebound in spite of their health challenges, as described in the resilience framework. In addition, both women had met goals specific to them, which they described as having a strong impact on their emotional and physical function. This is a demonstration of behavioral activation within the CAPABLE interventions.

CAPABLE addresses the functional and activity goals that low-income older adults seek to achieve, such as going to church, bathing themselves without help, and preparing food. We have shown that achieving these "small" changes can make big differences in outcomes of value to older adults themselves and to society, including hospital and nursing home use.[18] In the quotes below, two participants explained how CAPABLE helped them remain in their homes:

No one trains you to get old . . . you get trained as a kid, an adolescent and an adult . . . but no one helps you think about how to stay in your home as long as possible. . . . CAPABLE can help you with this. Things you never even think about. Count the number of steps, get involved in your community and let them know you're aging, think about what you need to do now to stay in your home when you're eighty and start working on this. (Male, 70 years old)

Before I started CAPABLE, I was going to check myself into a nursing home but since you all have been coming out to see me, I'm going to stay home! CAPABLE has helped me mentally and physically. (Female, 85 years old)

The CAPABLE program has shown consistent and promising results in each of the following three studies. Starting with a pilot trial of forty participants, then a one-armed trial funded by the Center for Medicare and Medicaid Innovation, and finally a definitive randomized control trial, CAPABLE has improved ADL ability in 75 percent of participants.[19] From start to finish, the average participant in CAPABLE starts with difficulty in four ADLs and finishes with difficulty in two areas. This improvement in two ADL areas is clinically and economically meaningful.[20] CAPABLE has also consistently decreased depressive symptoms. These are important outcomes for older adults and also for the health systems in which they are users.[21] The cost of the intervention is less than $3,000 per participant, yet evaluators from the Center for Medicare and Medicaid Services have shown it is associated with at least $30,000 in savings *per participant* over two years ($20,000 in Medicare costs over two years and $10,000 in Medicaid costs in one year).[22] Together, if replicated, that could mean $27,000 in savings for $3,000 spent for any one older adult living at home with a functional disability. The medical savings are due to decreased hospitalizations, rehospitalizations, and nursing home admissions. CAPABLE has grown from a pilot test to a randomized controlled trial to scaling in twenty cities in eleven states within eight years based on its ability to simultaneously help people age in place and decrease unnecessary medical use.

Here is a case example that illustrates how CAPABLE works to support older adults to meet their goals. Mr. D. is a sixty-four-year-old veteran who uses a wheelchair and walker for mobility. He has end-stage renal disease, which means his kidneys have failed in their ability to cleanse his blood, and he therefore goes for a dialysis treatment for three hours at a time, three days a week. He returns from these sessions exhausted, and, as the toxins in his blood build up until before the next session in two days, he becomes increasingly fatigued. He is a military veteran with multiple areas of pain from arthritis. Mr. D. has a stony facial expression and takes little pleasure in his usual activities.

At his first CAPABLE visit, he described this situation and determined that his functional goals were to work on his pain and on his strength/balance, reach things on the floor, shave standing up, and go outside on his own. He did not seek to address his mood. Over the course of the visits with the occupational therapist (OT) and the registered nurse (RN), he used the CAPABLE exercises based on Otago fall prevention; he now scoots with his legs in his wheelchair and can briefly stand. The CAPABLE handyperson installed a grab bar by his sink, and Mr. D. can now stand to shave, which makes him feel he can take care of himself with dignity. For pain, he uses the same CAPABLE exercises, a TENS (transcutaneous electrical nerve stimulation) unit, and a knee brace, all of which give him a bit of relief and together are quite effective. Toward the end of the CAPABLE program, he is smiling during our visits and not as fatigued after dialysis, so he can engage in evening activities, which also helps brighten his mood. He had not wanted to work directly on his mood, but these changes have improved his outlook. Prior to engaging with CAPABLE, his favorite activity was to go out onto his back porch, but someone had to hoist him up the small set of stairs. With several strategically placed grab bars and his new strength, he can get onto his back porch himself, without help, and enjoy himself.

We learned a number of lessons from this case:

1. CAPABLE staff should identify an individual's favorite activity. They should ask how the person pursued this activity in the past and what barriers have arisen to prevent his or her engaging in it. These barriers may be physical, financial, or social—many of which are fixable. Regardless of the caregiver's background or discipline, chances are that talking to the individual will result in appealing ideas and sustainable goals.
2. Older adults are resilient at any point in their health trajectory until the last few weeks of life. At first glance and from a medical perspective, Mr. D. might have seemed hopeless—a depressed man in constant pain and with limited mobility who was tethered to a kidney machine for much of his week and too exhausted to do much more than undergo dialysis. But by assessing Mr. D. for small functional goals, from both an OT and an RN perspective, as well as building up his home environment, Mr. D.'s home *and* his state of mind were transformed.
3. Pain and motivation are closely interconnected. Pain can be debilitating and keep people from engaging in activities they enjoy. The body's natural response to pain is to decrease stimuli in order to prevent pain, resulting in decreased activity. Less activity often leads to less flexibility and mobility, physiological responses to pain that can lead to depressive symptoms. The cycle of pain, loss of motivation, and depression can be one from which it is difficult to escape. The

CAPABLE nurse and OT use behavioral activation to provide motivation that can help a person break this cycle. With this motivation, the person can strive to meet pain goals, which may also help alleviate accompanying depressive symptoms.

As the population ages, the implications of the CAPABLE program become more important. Extending the amount of time older people can stay in their homes has multiple benefits, including increasing their ability to care for extended family members such as grandchildren and their ability to continue contributing to the community, which is important, as older adults are our fastest-growing natural resource.[23] CAPABLE targets the 40 percent of older adults who have difficulty with one or more ADLs. As the older population doubles in the next forty years, the number of individuals facing these challenges will likely multiply due to aging with obesity and other chronic conditions.

As we have demonstrated in this chapter, physical and social function are modifiable factors whose amelioration can improve the health, community participation, and ability to age in place of older adults. This is true even though there are currently large disparities in the health of the current cohort of older adults. Using theoretically based person-centered interventions is an ideal way to improve these key health indicators. The CAPABLE program has made a significant impact on the social and physical functioning of older adults.

The spread of the CAPABLE program to multiple health systems and its acceptance through different payment mechanisms testify to its common-sense approach and robust evidence base. There is a tremendous opportunity to improve the lives of current and future older adults through a person-centered approach that takes into account individual experiences and needs and helps older adults improve their social and physical functioning across various domains.

As we face a growing population of older adults, we will strengthen families, workers, communities, and economies if we decrease health disparities in the very cohort that most benefits from the advantages of aging in place. Strategies such as CAPABLE, based on dignity, behavioral activation, goal setting, and physical supports in the environment, can lead the way to this inclusive vision.

Notes

1. Theresa A. Keenan, *Home and Community Preferences of the 45+ Population* (Washington, DC: AARP, 2010), http://assets.aarp.org/rgcenter/general/home-community-services-10.pdf.

2. Ishani Ganguli, Jeffrey Souza, J. Michael McWilliams, and Ateev Mehrotra, "Trends in Use of the US Medicare Annual Wellness Visit, 2011–2014," *Journal of the American Medical Association* 317, no. 21 (June 2017): 2233–35.

3. Patrick L. Remington, Bridget B. Catlin, and Keith P. Gennuso, "The County Health Rankings: Rationale and Methods," *Population Health Metrics* 13, no. 11 (April 2015), https://doi.org/10.1186/s12963-015-0044-2.

4. Ibid.

5. Peter W. Greenwald, Michael E. Stern, Tony Rosen, Sunday Clark, and Neal Flomenbaum, "Trends in Short-Stay Hospitalizations for Older Adults from 1990 to 2010: Implications for Geriatric Emergency Care," *American Journal of Emergency Medicine* 32, no. 4 (April 2014): 311–14; Martin J. Prince, Fan Wu, Yanfei Guo, Luis M. Gutierrez Robledo, Martin O'Donnell, Richard Sullivan, and Salim Yusuf, "The Burden of Disease in Older People and Implications for Health Policy and Practice," *Lancet* 385, no. 9967 (February 2015): 549–62; Evelien E. S. van Riet, Arno W. Hoes, Kim P. Wagenaar, Alexander Limburg, Marcel A. J. Landman, and Frans H. Rutten, "Epidemiology of Heart Failure: The Prevalence of Heart Failure and Ventricular Dysfunction in Older Adults over Time—A Systematic Review," *European Journal of Heart Failure* 18, no. 3 (January 2016): 242–52; Meghan Warren, Kathleen J. Ganley, and Patricia S. Pohl, "The Association between Social Participation and Lower Extremity Muscle Strength, Balance, and Gait Speed in US Adults," *Preventive Medicine Reports* 4, no. 1 (December 2016): 142–47.

6. Sherry R. Glazier, John Schuman, Esther Keltz, Ashnor Vally, and Richard H. Glazier, "Taking the Next Steps in Goal Ascertainment: A Prospective Study of Patient, Team, and Family Perspectives Using a Comprehensive Standardized Menu in a Geriatric Assessment and Treatment Unit," *Journal of the American Geriatrics Society* 52, no. 2 (February 2004): 284–89; Elbert S. Huang, Rita Gorawara-Bhat, and Marshall H. Chin, "Self-Reported Goals of Older

Patients with Type 2 Diabetes Mellitus," *Journal of the American Geriatrics Society* 53, no. 2 (February 2005): 306–11.

7. Monika Ardelt, "Disentangling the Relations between Wisdom and Different Types of Well-being in Old Age: Findings from a Short-Term Longitudinal Study," *Journal of Happiness Studies* 17, no. 5 (October 2016): 1963–84; Dan P. McAdams, "The Positive Psychology of Adult Generativity: Caring for the Next Generation and Constructing a Redemptive Life," in *Positive Psychology*, ed. Jan D. Sinnott (New York: Springer, 2013), 191–205; Angela Schoklitsch and Urs Baumann, "Generativity and Aging: A Promising Future Research Topic?," *Journal of Aging Studies* 26, no. 3 (August 2012): 262–72.

8. Sarah L. Szanton and Jessica M. Gill, "Facilitating Resilience Using a Society-to-Cells Framework: A Theory of Nursing Essentials Applied to Research and Practice," *Advances in Nursing Science* 33, no. 4 (October 2010): 329–43.

9. Ibid.

10. Ibid.

11. Sheung-Tak Cheng, Emily P. M. Mak, Rosanna W. L. Lau, Natalie S. S. Ng, and Linda C. W. Lam, "Voices of Alzheimer Caregivers on Positive Aspects of Caregiving," *Gerontologist* 56, no. 3 (June 2016): 451–60, and Margaret E. Hughes, "A Strengths Perspective on Caregiving at the End-of-Life," *Australian Social Work* 68, no. 2 (November 2014): 156–68.

12. Michael Marmot, "The Influence of Income on Health: Views of an Epidemiologist," *Health Affairs* 21, no. 2 (March/April 2002): 31–46; Tracy Epton, Peter R. Harris, Rachel Kane, Guido M. van Koningsbruggen, and Paschal Sheeran, "The Impact of Self-Affirmation on Health-Behavior Change: A Meta-analysis," *Health Psychology* 34, no. 3 (March 2015): 187–96, and Emily B. Falk, Matthew Brook O'Donnell, Christopher N. Cascio, Francis Tinney, Yoona Kang, Matthew D. Lieberman, Shelley E. Taylor, Lawrence An, Kenneth Resnicow, and Victor J. Strecher, "Self-Affirmation Alters the Brain's Response to Health Messages and Subsequent Behavior Change," *Proceedings of the National Academy of Sciences* 112, no. 7 (February 2015): 1977–82.

13. Barbara Starfield, "Is Patient-Centered Care the Same as Person-Focused Care?," *Permanente Journal* 15, no. (Spring 2011): 63–69.

14. Pim Cuijpers, Annemieke van Straten, and Lisanne Warmerdam, "Behavioral Activation Treatments of Depression: A Meta-analysis," *Clinical Psychology Review* 27, no. 3 (May 2007): 318–26, and Kathleen D. Lyons, Ingrid A. Svensborn, Alice B. Kornblith, and Mark T. Hegel, "A Content Analysis of Functional Recovery Strategies of Breast Cancer Survivors," *The Occupational Therapy Journal of Research: Occupation, Participation and Health* 35, no. 2 (April 2015): 73–80.

15. Lyons et al., "A Content Analysis of Functional Recovery Strategies of Breast Cancer Survivors."

16. Laura N. Gitlin, Walter W. Hauck, Marie P. Dennis, Laraine Winter, Nancy Hodgson, and Sandy Schinfeld, "Long-Term Effect on Mortality of a Home Intervention that Reduces Functional Difficulties in Older Adults: Results from a Randomized Trial," *Journal of the American Geriatrics Society* 57, no. 3 (March 2009): 476–81, and Laura N. Gitlin, Laraine Winter, Marie P. Dennis, Mary Corcoran, and Walter W. Hauck, "A Randomized Trial of a Multicomponent Home Intervention to Reduce Functional Difficulties in Older Adults," *Journal of the American Geriatrics Society* 54, no. 5 (May 2006): 809–16.

17. Sarah L. Szanton, J. W. Wolff, B. Leff, Roland James Thorpe Jr., Elizabeth K. Tanner, C. Boyd, Q. Xue, J. Guralnik, David Bishai, Laura N. Gitlin, "CAPABLE Trial: A Randomized Controlled Trial of Nurse, Occupational Therapist and Handyman to Reduce Disability among Older Adults: Rationale and Design," *Contemporary Clinical Trials* 38, no. 1 (May 2014): 102–12.

18. Sarah Ruiz, Lynne Page Snyder, Christina Rotondo, Caitlin Cross-Barnet, Erin Murphy Colligan, and Katherine Giuriceo, "Innovative Home Visit Models Associated with Reductions in Costs, Hospitalizations, and Emergency Department Use," *Health Affairs* 36, no. 3 (March 2017): 425–32, and Sarah L. Szanton, Y. Natalia Alfonso, Bruce Leff, Jack Guralnik, Jennifer L. Wolff, Ian Stockwell, Laura N. Gitlin, David Bishai, "Medicaid Cost Savings of a Preventive Home Visit Program for Disabled Older Adults," *Journal of the American Geriatrics Society* 66, no. 3 (March 2018): 614–20.

19. The pilot trial of forty participants is described in Sarah L. Szanton, Roland J. Thorpe, Cynthia Boyd, Elizabeth K. Tanner, Bruce Leff, Emily Agree, Qian-Li Xue, Jerilyn K. Allen, Christopher L. Seplaki, Carlos O. Weiss, Jack M. Guralnik, and Laura N. Gitlin, "Community Aging in Place, Advancing Better Living for Elders: A Bio-Behavioral-Environmental Intervention to Improve Function and Health-Related Quality of Life in Disabled Older Adults," *Journal of the American Geriatrics Society* 59, no. 12 (December 2011): 2314–20. The one-armed trial funded by the Center for Medicare and Medicaid Innovation is described in Sarah L. Szanton, Bruce Leff, Jennifer L. Wolff, Laken Roberts, and Laura N. Gitlin, "Home-Based Care Program Reduces Disability and Promotes Aging in Place," *Health Affairs* 35, no. 9 (September 2016): 1558–63. Szanton, Leff, et al. are currently preparing a manuscript describing the definitive randomized control trial.

20. Szanton, Leff, "Home-Based Care Program Reduces Disability and Promotes Aging in Place"; Szanton, Alfonso, et al., "Medicaid Cost Savings of a Preventive Home Visit Program for Disabled Older Adults."

21. Lisa Alecxih, Sophie Shen, Iris Chan, Duke Taylor, and John Drabek, *Individuals Living in the Community with Chronic Conditions and Functional Limitations: A Closer Look,* The Lewin Group, January 2010, https://aspe.hhs.gov/system/files/pdf/75961/closerlook.pdf.

22. Ruiz et al., "Innovative Home Visit Models Associated with Reductions in Costs, Hospitalizations, and Emergency Department Use."

23. Erik H. Erikson, *The Life Cycle Completed: A Review* (New York: W. W. Norton, 1982).

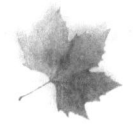

CHAPTER TEN

From Diagnosis to Person-Focused Prognosis
Toward a Healthy Political Economy of Aging in America

JUSTIN MUTTER

"The White Coats Are Coming," he announced with a wry smile. A fitting title for his book, I thought, but then I found myself looking down at my own white coat, wishing I hadn't worn it to my clinic today. Noticing my discomfort, he added kindly, "Well, I'll have to write a different . . . thingy . . . for you." I breathed an inaudible sigh of relief and smiled back. I was off the hook. Maybe. When Tom, as I will call him, said "thingy," he meant "another chapter in my book," but in the course of trying to speak, he had been unable to find the right word.[1] He was fighting a condition known as primary progressive aphasia, most likely attributable to an early stage of dementia. Though he was gradually losing command of his words,

Tom had decided to write a book about his experience with the healthcare system. Not about to be sidelined by his illness, he had set a goal of finishing the book before further decline in language made it impossible. He had a story to tell.

The Political Economy of Diagnosis and the Eclipse of the Older Person

Tom's story is a familiar one. Faced with complex cognitive and psychological symptoms and increasingly unable to work, he had been sent from doctor to doctor, white coat to white coat. Tests were ordered. Lab samples were drawn, again and again. Neurological imaging was obtained, and even a spinal tap was performed. All of this yielded inconclusive results. Tom's clinical signs and symptoms were somewhat atypical. Neurologists thought the underlying cause was psychiatric; psychiatrists thought it was neurological. Because no one would offer him a clear diagnosis, he couldn't qualify for disability services. At 62—just when he had expected to be winding down a career and finalizing retirement plans—he instead found himself jobless, plagued by economic hardship. Not yet Medicare eligible, he had been paying an extraordinary monthly sum for two years to maintain his health insurance under the Consolidated Omnibus Reconciliation Act (better known to those who have had to seek recourse to it by its distressing acronym, COBRA). By the time I met him, Tom hadn't been back to see a doctor in nearly a year. Exhausted from being guided in different directions, his financial resources drained by a mountain of bills, he had decided to get off the medical map. But when his disorder progressed, he warily returned to the house of medicine.

An explanation of Tom's prototypical narrative can be found in Charles Rosenberg's well-known article from the early part of this century, "The Tyranny of Diagnosis."[2] Though primarily a social and cultural historian, Rosenberg purposefully chose a set of political metaphors for his account of diagnosis, noting that he could just as easily have called the article "Diagnosis Mediates an Invisible Revolution." In Rosenberg's view, the act of diagnosis in American medicine has become so narrowly biomedical, so myopically disease-centric, that it often eclipses other, more holistic medical activities, such as prognosis and healing. More broadly, it has become the house of medicine's constitution, with principles and practices so immutable and inalienable as to be nearly imperceptible to us.

There is an ongoing chicken-and-egg debate in the historiography of American medicine about the relationship between concepts and systems. Does the centrality of diagnosis in medical epistemology lead to a technology-driven political economy of testing and therapeutic intervention? In more practical terms, is the conceptual process that Rosenberg describes responsible for $150 million investments in proton-beam radiation for a tiny fraction of rare cancers? Or, conversely, does a capitalist medical-industrial complex directly engineer diagnosis at the center, itself defining and refining medical epistemology and nosology (the branch of medical science dealing with the classification of diseases)?

The historiography of modern American medicine is littered with testaments on both sides. Rosenberg himself—as evidenced by his comment that diagnosis *mediates* a revolution—is probably most firmly (though not exclusively) in the first camp. Others have claimed that without the rise of capitalistic practices in systems of American healthcare and public health during the middle decades of the twentieth century, biomedicine would not be nearly as dominant as it is today. In this view, perhaps best exemplified in the work of E. Richard Brown, powerful organizations like the Rockefeller Foundation (whose approach is arguably recapitulated today through institutions like the Bill and Melinda Gates Foundation) built systems that reified narrow biomedical engagements with disease, ultimately rendering such engagements profitable.[3] Writing in 1979, Brown insisted that the historical record plainly reveals that "the major groups and forces that shaped the medical system sowed the seeds of the crisis we now face. The medical profession and other medical interest groups each tried to make medicine serve their own narrow economic and social interests."[4] A more contemporary correlate of this argument is often made by historians and sociologists of Alzheimer's disease, who maintain that Alzheimer's could not be codified as a diagnostic entity until federal research dollars were systematically applied to its study.[5] Political economy, in this account, mediates diagnosis.

In this chapter I argue that the history and science of aging in America reveal that both sides of the debate are germane. Since at least 1965, with the creation of Medicare as an insurance scheme for older adults, the political economy of aging has developed using an epistemology and financing system that are inextricably intertwined. Consequently, Tom does not distinguish between the diagnostic preoccupations of his healthcare providers and the system that augments those preoccupations. Rather, he experiences it all as an indivisible process from which his personal care needs are systematically sidelined. Following Rosenberg with a twist, in what follows I will refer to Tom's prototypical experience with American healthcare as an effect of the "political economy of diagnosis." Despite several merits, chiefly its ability to harness extraordinary technological power, the political economy of diagnosis is deeply flawed. It is flawed because it was built on a foundation with diagnosis as its cornerstone. Nowhere are its flaws more apparent than in the care of aging Americans, many of whom, like Tom, are struggling with advanced chronic illnesses.

The litany of public and private concerns about healthcare for older adults is well known: poor health outcomes, runaway costs, and inefficient and impersonal services. The mediocre state of our current care of older adults derives from two closely connected historical developments. The first is that, since its inception, Medicare's fiscal organization has relied almost exclusively on the political economy of diagnosis. The second is that this reliance has, ironically, largely ignored the evolving science of aging. Over time, insurance benefits have been narrowly construed as associated with specific disease entities. This reductionist turn has rendered Medicare payment policy at odds with older adults in the evening of their lives. Therefore, what we do for older adults in modern medicine often diverges substantially from who older adults are, and what they need. In the political economy of diagnosis, the disease eclipses the whole person. As Rosenberg writes, an individual "becomes visible to the health care system when diagnosed with an acute ailment but then returns to invisibility once that episode has been managed."[6]

In exploring the relationship between historical political economy and the modern science of aging, I aim to augment ongoing discourses about aging in America. There is a tendency in both health policy and academic discussions to view the current crisis in caring for older adults as a problem of demography or, perhaps, as the result of our cultural obsession with youth. So Lawrence Samuel, in his recent cultural history of aging, sees America's current predicament as a consequence of persistent ageism, which will, however, eventually be overpowered by the "gray power" of the Baby Boomer generation.[7] Other political histories of aging and healthcare trace a chronological, slowly unraveling "history of neglect" by which older adults have been relegated to the sidelines of modern urban economies and continue to struggle to make their voices heard. What Laura Olson in 1982 termed the "liberal accommodationist" view of modern aging—in which political forces must incrementally "compensate for the shortcomings of deficient institutions and reform particular public programs"—is alive and well in our time.[8] Yet, in her expansive account of the political economy of aging up until that time, Olson offers a narrative that is equally reductionist, in which aging has been entirely subject to capitalist ideology. In her description, the various programs of the Older Americans Act of 1965 have "buttress[ed] the power of financial institutions and support[ed] corporate practices."[9]

While there is merit in all of these accounts, together they tend to obviate a more expansive view of the political economy of aging in America, one capable of attending to myriad actors across state, capital, and other pertinent institutions. In her relentless focus on the federal government and capitalist ideology, for example, Olson declines to consider the role that medical education or Medicare administrative practices has played in the care of older adults. Drawing heavily from historical methodology in the political economy of health and disease, I contend that our current crisis in the care of older adults is not an accidental byproduct of demographic, epidemiologic, or ageist cultural phenomena but rather a holistic system by design. An account of the political economy of diagnosis will show that the past, present, and future of living with advanced illness in old age is "inseparable from the total history of communal organization and the economy."[10]

The Medicalization of "Benefits" as Diagnoses: Medicare and the Currency of Aging

Medicare has, of course, been the subject of widespread policy debate ever since it was signed into law as an amendment to the Social Security Act in

1965. But in 1983, the mood among policymakers and healthcare regulators across the nation was one of cautious optimism. In April of that year, President Ronald Reagan signed into law HR 1900 (Public Law 98-21). Unlike other major pieces of legislation involving America's healthcare system, Public Law 98-21 did not carry a catchy title proclaiming its commitment to "care" or to "health." It was simply known as "The Social Security Amendments of 1983," and its primary statutory focus was on the fiscal solvency of Social Security payments at a time of economic recession. As political scientist Rick Mayes describes the moment, "The most significant change in health policy since Medicare and Medicaid's passage in 1965 went virtually unnoticed by the general public."[11]

The amendments established a novel approach to Medicare payment known as the "prospective payment system" (PPS). Previously, Medicare—which was, from the outset, oriented primarily toward taxpayer funding for hospital services—had paid hospital systems retrospectively. Payments were organized, quite literally and straightforwardly, through a "cost plus" system, with disbursements covering a combination of the "reasonable" amount as designated by provider groups plus the cost of nursing care and hospital capital expenses.[12] In its earliest phase, Medicare ceded authority to physicians to determine which services were "reasonable and necessary," as the statute read, and what they should cost. Physicians rapidly became the "bedside bureaucrats" of government-funded healthcare for older adults.[13] Not surprisingly, the cost of providing hospital care exploded, often rising to three and four times the rate of inflation annually.

The PPS was a dramatic shift in payment policy, tying all hospital payments to "diagnosis-related groups" (DRGs). This system remains in effect today and has, to varying degrees, significantly influenced Medicare fiscal policy for outpatient care, as well as private insurance schemes. Effectively, rather than pay whatever costs hospitals happened to incur on a per diem basis, in 1983 the entity that runs Medicare, now known as the Centers for Medicare and Medicaid Services, resolved to pay expected universal charges for specific diagnoses or types of diagnoses. The disease entity became the locus of financial standardization and bureaucratization of claims data across the nation. In other words, the diagnostic classification of diseases was now the official currency for the political economy of healthcare for older adults.

There is continuing debate over the degree to which the PPS and DRGs have successfully controlled costs; nearly a decade after PPS implementation, hospital costs per person were still more than double what they were at the inception of the rule.[14] Yet for all of the scholarly discussion of its macroeconomic impact, the consequences of the PPS for the entire political economy of Medicare—as experienced by its beneficiaries—have largely been ignored. This neglect is due in part to a common half-truth narrative about the history of Medicare. It goes something like this: The establishment of Medicare in 1965 was based on a "politics of consensus" in which, after decades of inertia, a tenuous compromise between policymakers and shareholders of the nascent medical-industrial complex allowed insurance coverage for the geriatric population to move forward.[15]

Yet because this compromise was insecure, it had to be renegotiated over time. The philosophy behind sustaining it was "incrementalism," what political scientist Lawrence Jacobs celebrates as a peculiarly American "modesty and self-restraint borne out of respect for enduring structural limitations facing health reform."[16] An incrementalist approach to Medicare has, over several decades, led to gradually increasing benefits tempered by cost-control measures in a methodical process like the oscillation of a pendulum. In this account, a substantial shift in payment policy like that represented by the PPS—albeit one that retained a powerful role for medical providers to set the terms for pricing—was an unavoidable rung on the health policy ladder that Americans have been climbing since the New Deal.

The problem with the narrative of incremental inevitability is that it neglects at least two critical features of the decision to link Medicare fiscal policy to DRGs. First, alternatives *were* available. As evidenced by federal interest in capitation and managed care in the 1990s, per diem payments did not have to be linked primarily to specific diagnoses. In fact, at the time of its enactment, the PPS was not even well studied as a viable policy option. Having originated as a means for data collection, it had been briefly tested as fiscal policy in only one state (New Jersey), and the first major research paper to assess its impact in that state would not be published until 1986. The results were underwhelming: "It is a system," the authors concluded, "that invites cost shifting before cost saving."[17] Viewed in its proper historical context, the PPS was more a policy fad than a carefully considered, gradualist strategy.

Second, while the story of incrementalist fiscal policy in Medicare pays close attention to political discourse, it overlooks the broader economic changes resulting from incremental reform, changes that had a dramatic impact on older adults' experience of both healthy and unhealthy aging. While the policy may have been gradualist, its effects were anything but gradual. Medicare was a powerful catalyst for medical specialization in America, as well as for the rapid expansion of biotechnology and biomedical research.[18] This was in no small part due to Medicare's financial support for care and capital expenses generated by hospitals. Medicare payments alone may have generated over a third of national hospital growth in the program's early years.[19] Acute, episodic, and high-technology medicine based in hospitals rapidly became the center of activity in the American healthcare system. What's more, the advent of DRGs meant that these activities themselves revolved around an axis of diagnosis. As Rosenberg notes at the end of his history of American hospitals, this model has meant that "disease does not exist unless it can be coded."[20] The history of Medicare fiscal policy shows that diagnostic coding is *the* mechanism by which diseases are recognized, and *therefore paid for*, by the healthcare system. Diagnosis is not just a professional and social act; it is a financial one.

Historians Carole Haber and Brian Gratton have argued convincingly that, in contrast to one-dimensional historiographic notions that Social Security benefits reversed a trend of industrialization, lifting millions of older adults out of poverty, more accurately it *redistributed* social and financial responsibility for retirement.[21] Whereas prior to Social Security the experience of retirement was conditioned by family, community, and workplace resources, Social Security rendered it more prominently contingent on the state. A similar argument could be made for Medicare, which was, of course, originally conceived as a subdivision of Social Security. By codifying the political economy of diagnosis, Medicare has been a major engine of the medical-industrial complex, molding the experiences of older adults throughout the healthcare system in the late twentieth and early twenty-first centuries.

Medicare's use of diagnoses as the currency of the state, however, has engendered a conflict that is often underappreciated. It has pitted older adults' financial security against their health. While an older adult living with multiple advanced illnesses may take comfort in Medicare's commitment to covering novel treatments, hospitalizations, and other highly specialized care, it is unclear whether these interventions translate into salutary, person-centered outcomes. Health economists Amy Finkelstein and Robin McKnight, for example, maintain that while out-of-pocket spending on healthcare among older adults significantly decreased during Medicare's first decade, insurance benefits had no measurable impact on mortality during that time.[22] A more contemporary analysis has questioned the previously held assumption that Medicare coverage for adults who were formerly without insurance has improved health outcomes.[23]

While these economic analyses remain matters of debate, the fact that Medicare's relative efficacy is under scrutiny should come as no surprise. During its fifty-two-year history, decisions about insurance benefits have been driven primarily by fiscal concerns and executed through the political economy of diagnosis. This is Medicare's core weakness. As economist Uwe Reinhardt noted at Medicare's fiftieth anniversary, "The flaw in the DRG system lies in its basis on what are actually *relative costs* incurred in producing the various DRG cases, rather than on the *relative value* to patients or to society as a whole of the services covered by the DRGs."[24] The concept of value is teleological; it requires us to formulate a positive vision of health for older adults rather than respond to negative concerns about the cost of services provided.

The political economy of diagnosis disseminated through Medicare benefits is incommensurate, in many ways, with the health needs of older adults, particularly those with multiple biopsychosocial concerns. The evolution of this trend in American healthcare reflects a subtype of medicalization distinct from Peter Conrad's classic formulation, according to which "medical jurisdiction" widens its hold on social problems previously considered to be "nonmedical."[25] Health insurance benefits can hardly be characterized as nonmedical problems. Yet when healthcare services must be tied to specific diagnoses in order for providers or recipients to be reimbursed, human health is no longer an indivisible, whole-person phenomenon. The regime of diagnosis is thoroughly reductionist, opting to build systems of fractured transactions rather than aim for a unifying mission of well-being. This is a kind of medicalization by means of biomedical atomization, a social process that recasts human health as a mere sum of its parts.

The Meeting of the Science of Geriatrics with the Political Economy
of Diagnosis in the Evening of Life

Biomedical atomization works well, and in some cases superbly, for several aspects of modern healthcare. Individual diseases can be identified and cured or effectively controlled. Targeted technologies and pharmacotherapies can alleviate symptoms and suffering. Yet the more complex one's problems and care, the less efficacious does the political economy of diagnosis become. Tom's story is a case in point. His experiences are typical of a widening gap between the science of caring for older adults and the healthcare services actually provided to them. In this section I explore this gap by reviewing the vanguard of clinical and scientific research in geriatric medicine and gerontology. My argument is twofold: first, that among older adults with multiple health problems and functional limitations, care is efficacious only if it is directed at the whole person rather than individual disease entities; and second, that the science of geriatric health policy correspondingly shows that only programs that approach older adults *as* whole persons tend to achieve what has been called the "Triple Aim" of better care, with improved satisfaction with services at lower cost.[26] The political economy of diagnosis, however, neglects precisely these holistic programs, setting the stage for an underperforming healthcare system.

There are two core advances in the science of aging that illuminate this gap. The first derives from clinical research in geriatric medicine, the second from health policy research in care systems for older adults. The first advance we might call the *functional imperative*. Although its earliest formulation dates back to Ignatz Leo Nascher's classic 1914 work *Geriatrics: The Diseases of Old Age and Their Treatment*, the functional imperative has seen expansive elucidation in recent decades. We now understand that in order to care successfully for older adults with chronic illnesses, we must work to heal the *whole person* as a mechanism for treating specific diseases. Healing the whole person necessarily requires a focus on global function: Are older persons able to function well in their current environment? What limitations do they have? What detriments to quality of life and well-being exist, and how might we overcome them?

Geriatric medicine is a practice attuned especially to these questions. As Mary Tinetti notes, geriatrics has evolved into a "metadiscipline," offering a set of insights and principles about health, illness, and well-being in older adults that is applicable to a wide variety of medical specialties, to public health, and to social services.[27] These insights and principles do *not*, however, depend on chronological age. Geriatrics is focused on older adults living with multiple health problems, with functional impairments including cognitive difficulties, and with complex biopsychosocial needs. In short, its scope primarily includes those living in the evening of life, at whatever age.

Over the past two decades, geriatric and gerontological researchers have, out of the functional imperative, delineated what is arguably the most important concept in the care of older adults: frailty syndrome. One should note that there is an important difference between a *geriatric* syndrome and the commonplace definition of a syndrome used in biomedical education. Students in the health professions are taught that a "syndrome" is a collection of symptoms that can be traced to a single cause. For example, trainees learn about Sjögren's syndrome, which is attributable to a distinct autoimmune process, or Marfan's syndrome, which is caused by a rare genetic disorder. In the care of older adults, however, a syndrome is something quite different. A geriatric syndrome has both multiple causes and complex effects, and therefore it must be approached with attention to the whole person.[28]

Frailty syndrome in older adults is a dynamic condition with many possible causes both inside and outside the body. A helpful working definition characterizes frailty as a condition of increased vulnerability to stressors, whether biological, psychological, or socioeconomic, due to a "decline in physiologic reserve and function."[29] This may or may not be related to processes of normal aging. We can think of functional assessment of older adults as a unique set of glasses we put on to be able to clearly view frailty along its spectrum. Where one falls along this spectrum depends on his or her relative vulnerability versus resilience in response to stressors. The critical point about frailty syndrome is that it is impossible to approach with a reductionist lens. Function is complex, broad, and dynamic. It requires consideration of one's environment, one's resources, and one's health concerns.

To illustrate the importance of frailty and function and to connect this to the second major advance in the science of aging, consider the story of an older adult I will call Charlotte. Eighty years old, Charlotte lives alone, her husband having died five years ago. She has family nearby who visit frequently, but because poor vision prevents her from driving, she spends most of her time at home by herself. She loves her home, where she has lived for fifty years, and is an avid consumer of books and music. She has multiple health concerns, including severe heart problems, moderate kidney problems, arthritis, and depression. She has Medicare for insurance and historically had a middle-class income, but neither she nor her husband was able to save much for retirement. She takes fifteen different prescription medications and sees five different medical specialists regularly. Often lightheaded and consequently afraid of falling, she also requires assistance with housework because of her breathing difficulties and with grocery shopping because of her inadequate vision.

Because of her functional difficulties, which have a variety of causes, Charlotte has mild to moderate frailty syndrome. This makes her more vulnerable to certain stressors than are some others her age. For instance, with her multiple medications, difficulty walking, and lightheadedness, she is in danger of falling and breaking a hip. Because of her frailty and the fragmentation of her care across many medical providers, Charlotte is at high risk for further decline in function and quality of life. This is one of the most important insights from geriatric research into frailty: More than any single disease or condition, frailty syndrome places older adults in jeopardy of early death, extensive disability, increased dependence on healthcare, and escalating medical expenditures.[30]

Because frailty can be dynamic, Charlotte's goal is to receive comprehensive services that can improve her functional capacity. And in fact, her goal is remarkably consistent with advances in the study of which medical programs are best for older adults, my second point. Over the past few decades, research has consistently shown that programs and services that aim to enhance global function and reduce frailty, rather than simply addressing individual diagnoses, can dramatically outperform the status quo. Yet there is no pill or procedure to treat frailty syndrome. Just as frailty's causes are manifold, so must be the interventions to address it. What is striking about services that provide these interventions is that they at once improve health outcomes and reduce health expenditures. A recent demonstration program in Baltimore, for example, employed occupational therapists, nurses, and "handymen" to work together with low-income older adults to achieve their functional goals. This program rapidly became the most cost-saving project in the history of federal insurance coverage, nearly halving expenditures over a several-month period while augmenting participants' health. Similarly, small home-based care programs focused on holistic care for frail older adults have far outpaced large technocratic policy schemes like those offered by accountable care organizations in cost-effectiveness and care achievements.[31]

Yet Medicare's political economy of diagnosis rarely allows for these services. The two programs cited above, for instance, were financed for the short term in just a few cities by means of temporary grants outside the realm of traditional Medicare benefits. What Charlotte would welcome most urgently is this kind of comprehensive care, aimed at advancing her overall function and provided to her in her home. But that kind of service is difficult, if not impossible, to administer under the fiscal terms of Medicare's political economy of diagnosis.

Not surprisingly, because this regime fails to close the gap between the science of aging and services that older adults most need and desire, health outcomes for many older persons are poor. Consider those living with dementia, which is frequently accompanied by frailty syndrome. Healthcare costs for persons with dementia in the last five years of life come to around $300,000 and are nearly double that for people living with cancer or heart problems.[32] Despite these tremendous expenditures, quality of care and overall health outcomes for persons living with dementia are mediocre at best, largely because our diagnostic regime is incapable of conceptualizing frailty, much less responding to it appropriately. There is no DRG for this condition. Advanced frailty is now even explicitly disallowed as an admitting diagnosis for Medicare hospice services.[33] It barely exists in the eyes of Medicare payment policy.

Toward a Healthy Political Economy of Aging: Person-Focused Prognosis

The political economy of diagnosis is the house of medicine that we have built. Our current predicament in the care of older adults is not a problem of demography. It is not a side effect of industrial capitalism. It is not a byproduct of cultural ageism. While these phenomena are no doubt contributory, the fundamental problem with this house, beginning with its foundation, is its design. This design never included a positive, comprehensive vision of health for older adults approaching the ends of their lives. With such an incomplete design, it is no surprise that our house is now so ill-suited to those who enter it.

Since 1965, Medicare has been a fiscal program. It is not a health program for older adults. With decades of dissonance between the science of aging and the technologies of medical care to which Medicare beneficiaries have access, the political economy of diagnosis has conducted disharmony into the lives of older adults. In light of this dissonance, Medicare's interlocutors continue to worry that we remain beset by many of the same questions that arose soon after its inception.[34] The most important of these is simple but pivotal: how can we build a healthy political economy for older adults in the evening of their lives?

In this chapter I have contended that the first step to answering this question is to correctly identify the root of our problem. To extend the metaphor of the house of medicine, it is essential that we see the problem as foundational rather than one requiring a more superficial renovation. The historic and, to some degree, rhetorical power of the incrementalist political economy of diagnosis, however, leads even some of Medicare's staunchest critics to recommend what are in effect cosmetic repairs, doomed to fail. In his wide-ranging account of the history of Medicare administrative law and reform efforts, for example, Nicholas Bagley convincingly dissects the flaws in the very structure of Medicare, arguing that until Medicare can definitively influence the behaviors of medical providers at the bedside, its efficacy will be impaired. Yet in exposing the weaknesses of the Affordable Care Act's Medicare innovations, Bagley looks to processes for the direct regulation of medical providers' activities, what he calls "bring[ing] bureaucracy to the bureaucrats."[35] Similarly, physician Christine Cassel calls for the modernization of a program that was "developed in response to the prevailing healthcare needs of the elderly" at its inception.[36] Although Cassel rightly urges Medicare to create a renewed "social contract for health security" in addition to "income security," she fully embraces the policy tools of incrementalism: quality improvement, expansion of insurance benefits, care management, and other methodologies.[37]

These are valuable efforts, but if enacted alone, they will not restore the house of medicine for older adults. Checklists, quality metrics, and a myopic focus on fiscal policy are common features of what Lawrence Brown aptly terms Medicare's philosophy of "technocratic corporatism."[38] According to this philosophy, Medicare's flaws can be *managed* through greater efficiencies; however, its defining structure is overall sound. We need paint, sheetrock, and perhaps a reshuffling of furniture, but not a fresh foundation.

My exploration of the gap between Medicare's political economy of diagnosis and the science of aging, however, suggests that rationalized bureaucracy and technocracy will succeed only if regulation is guided by a person-centered mission. For older adults living with advanced illnesses, these technocratic efforts—many of them active today in healthcare systems across the nation—are like trying to drive "square pegs" into "round holes."[39] But it doesn't have to be this way. The examples of innovative, person-centered programs for older adults I have discussed prove the contrary. The science of aging and geriatric health policy shows unequivocally that our efforts can succeed if they are buttressed by a person-centered architecture.

It is not too difficult to imagine a health system for older adults in the evening of their lives that revolves around something other than diagnosis. We might call this a political economy of *prognosis*. If diagnosis asks, "What does this person have?," prognosis asks something quite different: "In view of the whole person—health, illness, vulnerabilities, and social supports—how is this person doing, what is her or his probable course, and how can we alter that course for the better?" In his history of technological medicine, Stanley Reiser pursues the answers to similar questions and comes to what he calls the "adaptive perspective" of health and illness, which has a rich lineage dating back to Greek medicine. The adaptive approach can "govern" the "structuralist" practices and technologies of diagnosis through relationships. For Reiser, relationships—between provider and patient, between patient and community, and between provider, patient, and society—are critical for dialogue and adjudication among healthcare's byzantine choices.[40] Prognosis can be this adaptive, relational guide in the care of older adults in the twenty-first century.

As a thought experiment, consider what might have happened if Tom had taken his concerns to a clinic governed by the political economy of prognosis. Tom, we recall, suffers from an early form of dementia that significantly alters his speech, a development that has, in turn, dramatically affected his functional capacities. Under a prognostic regime, Tom's healthcare provider would not be fixated on diagnostic codes but on how the symptoms of his illness were altering his health trajectory. Certainly his provider would have made use of reasonable diagnostic technologies in order to better assess the possible causes of his concerns, but Tom would not have been referred, and re-referred, to multiple specialists, seeking an "answer" for the better part of two years. Rather, because the responsibility of the provider would be to assist with Tom's prognosis as a whole person, a provisional diagnosis would likely have been offered. Due to his rapidly progressive functional difficulties and because diagnosis would not have been the key unlocking all benefits, Tom would have easily qualified for disability services and would not have seen his life's savings depleted by years of COBRA payments and medical bills. Tom would have received all he ever wanted from a health system: guidance and support. Knowing that his condition was likely incurable—but quite treatable—Tom would have received person-centered care in his home as his illness evolved. Perhaps he would even have had caregiver assistance to accomplish his primary goal of writing a book. And perhaps he would have decided to title his book not *The White Coats Are Coming* but *The White Coats Came—and Went*. All of this care would have been consistent with the best of the science of aging with advanced illness and, moreover, would have been considerably less expensive to provide than the medicalized benefits offered in the political economy of diagnosis.

All of this is easy to imagine because it is human and humane; it is what most of us would want for ourselves and for our loved ones. Of course, just because it is easy to imagine does not mean it is easy to build; nonetheless, a political economy of prognosis would certainly be no more difficult to construct than was our political economy of diagnosis. We just have to collectively commit to its architecture. There will be winners and losers in the new political economy, just as there are in our current one, albeit with an important difference: In the future, the delineation of those given a prominent role and those given a role on the sidelines will be made according to a teleological assessment of value: how best to support older adults in the evening of their lives. The good news is that this is already happening in many pockets of innovation around the United States. The task is to move it from pockets out into the open, accessible to all.

Notes

1. Patient narratives in this chapter are based on real experiences but have been significantly edited and adapted to protect the identity of the persons referenced.

2. Charles E. Rosenberg, "The Tyranny of Diagnosis: Specific Entities and Individual Experience," *Milbank Quarterly* 80, no. 2 (June 2002): 237–60.

3. E. Richard Brown, *Rockefeller Medicine Men: Medicine and Capitalism in America* (Berkeley: University of California Press, 1979). For more on parallels between the Rockefeller Foundation and the Gates Foundation, see, Anne-Emanuelle Birn, "Gates's Greatest Challenge: Transcending Technology as Public Health Ideology," *Lancet* 366, no. 9484 (March 2005): 514–19.

4. Brown, *Rockefeller Medicine Men*, 1.

5. Claudia Chaufan, Brooke Hollister, Jennifer Nazareno, and Patrick Fox, "Medical Ideology as a Double-Edged Sword: The Politics of Cure and Care in the Making of Alzheimer's Disease," *Social Science and Medicine* 74, no. 5 (March 2011): 788–95.

6. Rosenberg, "The Tyranny of Diagnosis," 255.

7. Lawrence R. Samuel, *Aging in America: A Cultural History* (Philadelphia: University of Pennsylvania Press, 2017), 165.

8. Laura K. Olson, *The Political Economy of Aging: The State, Private Power, and Social Welfare* (New York: Columbia University Press, 1982), 21.

9. Ibid., 216.

10. Steven Feierman, "Struggles for Control: The Social Roots of Health and Healing in Modern Africa," *African Studies Review* 28, nos. 2–3 (June–September 1985): 73–147, 73.

11. Rick Mayes, "The Origins, Development, and Passage of Medicare's Revolutionary Prospective Payment System," *Journal of the History of Medicine and Allied Sciences* 62, no. 1 (January 2007): 21–55, 21.

12. Karen Davis, Gerald Anderson, and Earl Steinberg, "Diagnosis-Related Group Prospective Payment: Implications for Health Care and Medical Technology," *Health Policy* 4, no. 2 (1984): 139–47.

13. Nicholas Bagley, "Bedside Bureaucrats: Why Medicare Reform Hasn't Worked," *Georgetown Law Journal* 101, no. 3 (2013): 519–80.

14. Stuart H. Altman and Donald A. Young, "A Decade of Medicare's Prospective Payment Program—Success or Failure?" *Journal of American Health Policy* 3, no. 2 (March–April 1993): 11–19.

15. Jonathan Oberlander, *The Political Life of Medicare* (Chicago: University of Chicago Press, 2003), 157.

16. Lawrence R. Jacobs, "The Medicare Approach: Political Choice and American Institutions," *Journal of Health Politics, Policy and Law* 32, no. 2 (April 2007): 159–86, 184.

17. William C. Hsiao, Harvey M. Sapolsky, Daniel L. Dunn, and Sanford L. Weiner, "Lessons of the New Jersey DRG Payment System," *Health Affairs* 5, no. 2 (Summer 1986): 32–45, 42.

18. Rosemary Stevens, *American Medicine and the Public Interest: A History of Specialization* (Berkeley: University of California Press, 1998).

19. Amy Finkelstein, "The Aggregate Effects of Health Insurance: Evidence from the Introduction of Medicare," *Quarterly Journal of Economics* 122, no. 1 (February 2007): 1–37.

20. Charles E. Rosenberg, *The Care of Strangers: The Rise of America's Hospital System* (Baltimore: Johns Hopkins University Press, 1995), 351.

21. Carole Haber and Brian Gratton, *Old Age and the Search for Security: An American Social History* (Bloomington, IN: Indiana University Press, 1994).

22. Amy Finkelstein and Robin McKnight, "What Did Medicare Do? The Initial Impact of Medicare on Mortality and Out of Pocket Medical Spending," *Journal of Public Economics* 92, no. 7 (July 2008): 1644–69.

23. Daniel Polsky, Jalpa A. Doshi, José Escarce, Willard Manning, Susan M. Paddock, Liyi Cen, and Jeannette Rogowski, "The Health Effects of Medicare for the Near-Elderly Uninsured," *Health Services Research* 44, no. 3 (June 2009): 926–45.

24. Uwe E. Reinhardt, "Medicare Innovations in the War over the Key to the US Treasury," in *Medicare and Medicaid at 50: America's Entitlement Programs in the Age of Affordable Care*, ed. Alan B. Cohen, David C. Colby, Keith Wailoo, and Julian E. Zelizer (New York: Oxford University Press, 2015), 176.

25. Peter Conrad, *The Medicalization of Society: On the Transformation of Human Conditions into Treatable Disorders* (Baltimore: Johns Hopkins University Press, 2007).

26. Donald M. Berwick, Thomas W. Nolan, and John Whittington, "The Triple Aim: Care, Health, and Cost," *Health Affairs* 27, no. 3 (May/June 2008): 759–69.

27. Mary Tinetti, "Mainstream or Extinction: Can Defining Who We Are Save Geriatrics?" *Journal of the American Geriatrics Society* 64, no. 7 (June 2016): 1400–1404.

28. Sharon K. Inouye, Stephanie Studenski, Mary E. Tinetti, and George A. Kuchel, "Geriatric Syndromes: Clinical, Research, and Policy Implications of a Core Geriatric Concept," *Journal of the American Geriatrics Society* 55, no. 5 (May 2007): 780–91.

29. Xujiao Chen, Genxiang Mao, and Sean X. Leng, "Frailty Syndrome: An Overview," *Clinical Interventions in Aging* 9, no. 1 (March 2014): 433–41.

30. Rebecca S. Crow, Matthew C. Lohman, Alexander J. Titus, Martha L. Bruce, Todd A. Mackenzie, Stephen J. Bartels, and John A. Batsis, "Mortality Risk along the Frailty Spectrum: Data from the National Health and Nutrition Examination Survey, 1999 to 2004," *Journal of the American Geriatrics Society* 66, no. 3 (March 2018): 496–502.

31. Sarah L. Szanton, Y. Natalia Alfonso, Bruce Leff, and Jack Guralnik, "Medicaid Cost Savings of a Preventive Home Visit Program for Disabled Older Adults," *Journal of the American Geriatric Society* 66, no. 3 (March 2018): 614–20; Sarah L. Szanton, Bruce Leff, Jennifer L. Wolff, Laken Roberts, and Laura N. Gitlin, "Home-Based Care Program Reduces Disability and Promotes Aging in Place," *Health Affairs* 35, no. 9 (September 2016): 1558–63; James Rotenberg, Bruce Kinosian, Peter Boling, and George Taler, "Home-Based Primary Care: Beyond Extension of the Independence at Home Demonstration," *Journal of the American Geriatrics Society* 66, no. 4 (February 2018): 812–17.

32. Amy S. Kelley, Kathleen McGarry, Rebecca Gorges, and Jonathan S. Skinner, "The Burden of Health Care Costs for Patients with Dementia in the Last Five Years of Life," *Annals of Internal Medicine* 163, no. 10 (November 2015): 729–36.

33. Vyjeyanthi S. Periyakoil, "Frailty as a Terminal Illness," *American Family Physician* 88, no. 6 (September 2013): 363–68.

34. Rosemary A. Stevens, "Health Care in the Early 1960s," *Health Care Financing Review* 18, no. 2 (Winter 1996): 11–22.

35. Bagley, "Bedside Bureaucrats," 566.

36. Christine K. Cassel, *Medicare Matters: What Geriatric Medicine Can Teach American Health Care* (Berkeley: University of California Press, 2005), 87.

37. Cassel, *Medicare Matters*, 213.

38. Lawrence D. Brown, "Technocratic Corporatism and Administrative Reform in Medicare," *Journal of Health Policy, Politics, and Law* 10, no. 3 (June 1985): 579–99.

39. Vyjeyanthi S. Periyakoil, "Square Pegs, Round Holes: Our Healthcare System is Failing Seriously Ill Older Adults in Their Last Years," *Journal of the American Geriatrics Society* 66, no. 1 (January 2018): 15–17.

40. Stanley Joel Reiser, *Technological Medicine: The Changing World of Doctors and Patients* (New York: Cambridge University Press, 2009), 186–203.

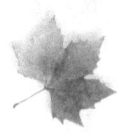

Conclusion

PAUL SCHERZ

The evening of life is a time of confusion, contention, and concern. From a societal perspective, there are clear practical problems in regard to supporting an aging demographic, especially given the ballooning medical expenses to pay for treatments of questionable benefit. Yet there are deeper cultural and existential problems that are suggested by epidemics of loneliness and anxiety among the aging. Despite mounting evidence of the scope of the problems we face in understanding how to age well, contemporary academic discourse offers few resources to help those approaching the evening of life either to live well or to help their lives go well. It is thus a site ripe for interdisciplinary cooperation in order to develop an ethics of aging.

As Joseph Davis argues in the first chapter, underlying all of these problems is the very amorphousness of old age in our society. There is no clearly defined cultural role for those who have passed retirement age. The social norms and roles of healthy middle age, themselves in the process of transformation because of the extension of adolescence, have expanded to colonize all of later life. Therefore, those in the evening of life seek to continue to exemplify the energy and virtues required of those in the prime of their working careers. Since continuing to fulfill such norms with an aging body becomes impossible at some point in the evening of life—earlier or later depending on one's luck and access to preventive health care—those in old age are destined to fail. Through this process, old age itself becomes devalued.

Even worse, the norms governing healthy middle age are themselves based on an illusion arising from liberal modernity's false picture of the person. In this conclusion I will discuss three areas in which contrasting understandings of aspects of human life have emerged as themes in the chapters of this volume: that in which persons are seen as self-optimizing versus dependent; that in which human temporality is understood as engaged in an open versus a closed future; and that in which the self is pictured as individual versus relational. The chapters collected here show how the second member of each pair embodies an understanding of the human that we must embrace if our culture is to recover a healthier picture of the evening of life. Moreover, these chapters suggest ways to adjust behaviors and structures to encourage these understandings of human life. Developing a better picture of the human is the first step toward recovering a cultural role for an old age that is seen as good in itself, which is necessary if we are to confront the practical problems facing us.

The Optimized Self and the Problem of Vulnerability

The vision of the person embedded in the successful aging movement is one of continual self-optimization. One must monitor and improve one's health (through exercise, yoga, and medication), one's cognition (through online games and other mental exercises), and one's productivity (through embarking on second careers). If one is not successful, if one succumbs to illness, dementia, or just a general decline in energy and activity, then one fails at aging. As Janelle Taylor and Joseph Davis point out, even if successful-aging advocates describe these shortcomings as normal aging, the opposite of success is failure.

These goals are not unique to later stages of life, of course, but are essential to the norms governing all of human life. From their preschool years, people must continually focus on developing their human, social, and monetary capital, as well as that of their children. If one is not constantly progressing, one is falling behind—children will not get into the right high school, which will lead to the right university, which will guarantee them the right entry-level job, which will put them on the ladder for jobs with ever-greater rewards of money and prestige, brilliant careers that are still shaded by the cloud of precarity. While all eras have had a measure of competitive striving, what is remarkable about our own is how early it starts—and that the treadmill never ends. To the end of life, one must constantly strive to achieve, if only in terms of fitness and activity.

Yet this ideal of continuous self-optimization is belied by the human condition. Goals of continuous success and achievement must be tempered by acknowledging that humans are creatures of vulnerability and dependency. The strength and independent drive necessary for this continual optimization will eventually fail through sickness, sadness, obstacles, or simply weariness, and then one's vulnerability to circumstances and one's reliance on others will be plain to see. This vulnerability is not a failing or an exceptional circumstance, but, as I noted in chapter 3, it is an essential part of being embodied creatures. As Bryan Turner argues, our failure to recognize this fact arises from the general failure in the social sciences to attend to the body. The body is vulnerable to illness and injury throughout life, but this vulnerability becomes especially apparent as the body ages. Narratives of continual self-optimization are possible only insofar as they ignore these facts.

The difficulty in developing this authentic understanding of the human arises not only from the extensive cultural pressures pushing pictures of active and fit older adults. It also arises from within the structures of medicine. The tyranny of diagnosis described by Justin Mutter means that if the body tires or weakens, there must be something specifically wrong with it. It cannot be that the body is merely aging, taking part in an entirely normal pattern of decline, a decline that should be slowed and dealt with as much as possible, but one that is the usual way of all flesh nonetheless. No, instead there must be an individual problem that is isolated and determined. It cannot be a general syndrome like frailty. Nor can care be based on the doctor's prognosis, which arises from long experience of engaging with the aging body. Medicine must find a specific diagnosis at the root of the general problems of vulnerability.

It is this blindness to the reality of the vulnerability of human embodiment that in part makes current narratives of the evening of life so inauthentic. While these narratives embrace a certain vision of authenticity in the form of being one's true self through achievement and exercise, Kevin Aho and Charles Guignon describe a much richer existentialist understanding of authenticity. In this understanding, true authenticity must be grounded in accepting the reality of one's situation. For those at the evening of life, this acceptance must include growing physical impairment in some form, though everyone at any stage of life should come to terms with the possibility of illness, death, and failure. The real achievement, in the Christian as well as many other traditions, is not the futile attempt to stave off this vulnerability, although it is reasonable to do what one can to stay healthy; rather, true success is growing in the humility, humor, generosity, and grace necessary to live as vulnerable creatures. It is an achievement that Wilfred McClay vividly describes through the narrative of his mother's life after a stroke.

These chapters offer many suggestions of how one can develop a more authentic existence. As Guignon argues, contemporary older adults need new narratives, or at least they should recover older narratives that allow for the vulnerabilities of old age. Rather than the stories of perpetual achievement portrayed in the media targeting older adults, contemporary society needs stories that prepare one for the acceptance of illness and decline. Rather than a narrative of the life course as one of unending capacity-building and achievement from the cradle onward, there needs to be a narrative that differentiates the various stages in life, giving each its place, but also allowing for an arc that connects these different stages. It is this narrative connectivity of life that allows us to see with McClay the face of former youth in the elderly and the possible face of old age in the young.

Further, society needs medical structures that allow for a picture of vulnerable old age. Part of this requires changes in the Medicare funding regime, as Mutter argues, through which care is not merely tied to diagnostic categories but can also respond to the needs suggested by a prognosis of the growing frailty of the aging body. As the CAPABLE program described by Sarah Szanton and Janiece Taylor shows, accepting the vulnerability of the aging body does not mean just abandoning it to decline. Accepting vulnerability means helping a person adapt to it and shaping the physical environment to respond to it, whether that means installing grab bars in the home or asking local authorities to create longer walk signals at surrounding traffic lights. It allows for a frank assessment of both the assets and the vulnerabilities that one has so that one can build on the assets and adjust for the vulnerabilities, allowing for as much continuing function as possible. An authentic picture of old age opens up other options for older adults beyond the youthful vitality of active gym-goers or the abandonment of those who fail to achieve this ongoing vitality in nursing homes. Instead, vulnerable bodies can be recognized and supported as far as possible.

Pictures of the Future

Contemporary understandings of aging are also affected by current stances toward temporality. As Davis and Aho suggest, people envision themselves as having an open and indefinite future. Life after retirement would seemingly stretch off into an almost endless future. This is of course an inaccurate picture of life. As the discussions of Heidegger in this volume suggest, the human future is closed by the horizon of death. All plans must be made with that horizon in mind. Yet our society hides this inevitable temporal closure.

Much has been written since Geoffrey Gorer's 1955 article "The Pornography of Death," on the hiddenness of contemporary dying.[1] Of course, end-of-life care has changed radically since the 1950s. With the explosion of writings arguing that people must be aware of death, from the death awareness movement to contemporary encouragements to prepare for death, one might suspect that the popular framing of death as silenced is rather like Foucault's discussion of Victorian taboos toward sex.[2] Foucault famously argued against the repressive hypothesis in regard to sexuality by showing that Victorians were constantly talking about sex, that the discourse surrounding sexuality in fact exploded in the Victorian era. Yet there still seems to be a hiddenness in the contemporary view of death. Few people fill out advanced directives.[3] Most popular discussions of death surround the need to eliminate it in the form of violent death and disease. And, unlike sex, few people have many experiences of death.

Contemporary dying still generally occurs in medical settings, far from the eyes of most people. People not working in medical or emergency settings will rarely see more than a couple of deaths over the course of their lives. Even the decline due to aging that presages death remains hidden, sequestered in nursing homes or in the lonely homes of individuals who can no longer engage in public life.

The structures of medical care reinforce the temporality of an open future. As Sharon Kaufman argues, all deaths are now considered premature. Thus all deaths are ones that could or should have been avoided.[4] The framing of medical decision-making renders the decision to forgo treatment, even a fairly invasive and difficult treatment like the implantation of a device in the heart or an organ transplant, almost impossible. Once Medicare reimburses such a treatment, it becomes the standard of care. A decision to reject such treatment thus is seen as rejecting standard treatment and dooming yourself or a relative to an early death. As many have remarked, the framework of medicine seemingly makes death a choice, thus making living indefinitely seem like a choice. In discussions of organ transplants, one seems to be able to choose whether one wants to add another ten years to one's life, thus pushing off one's consideration of the inevitable temporal closure of death.

This trust in an open future is a second form of our inauthentic existence. By ignoring death, one does not accept the truth of one's condition. It is a form of inauthenticity pushed upon the aging individual by advertisements, articles, popular self-help books, and the medical system itself. It prevents the evening of life from assuming its own proper form as the time when the limitations of the future become ever more pressing.

However, recognizing the failures of contemporary experiences of time opens up an avenue of hope by allowing a new relationship to time. As Aho argues, the realization that one's time on earth is not indefinite drives one to prioritize one's goals. The specter of death clears away distractions of pointless self-optimization in areas that are not important. More importantly, realizing that the future is not open can drive one to truly experience the present moment rather than seeing it merely as an instrumental resource to be used as a way to further future-directed goals. Instead one is open to the wonder that can be found in every instant, primed to fully enjoy what each moment can offer. Such a transformation of attention reframes the slowing-down of old age from merely an impediment to the swift achievement of future goals to an unwished-for grace that allows one to savor what the present offers. The sociological research cited by Turner suggests that many people in the evening of life may already have embraced these modified understandings of temporality, if only at a subconscious level, but an explicit engagement with them would help many more people.

In order to take full advantage of these insights into the temporal form of human life, changes must be made in the late modern shape of life. Some of these changes are tied to ceasing to view life as aimed at endless self-optimization, a stance toward life that drives one constantly toward the open future. Guignon notes that if one wishes to live reverently in old age, gratefully accepting what life and nature have to give, one needs to try to live more authentically in one's early years. One needs to attempt to form a steady outlook throughout the whole of life that resolutely accepts the temporal closure of death. In many cultures and traditions, an explicit preparation for death, including sets of exercises like the *memento mori*, ought to be undertaken from an early age if one wishes to live well. Paradoxically to our ears, in the past the young were encouraged to embrace the temporal stance toward the world, acknowledging one's limited future, which is most easily seen as one approaches old age. In Foucault's reading of Stoic ethics, the life of old age was a destination that one should seek, representing a culmination of a virtuous life.[5] Our society has completely reversed this relationship, encouraging the elderly to accept the temporal stance most natural to the young. It will thus take work for anyone to fully embrace this transformation of temporality.

The Relational Self

Of course this positive existentialist stance toward the temporality of old age is easier if one's life is fairly comfortable. It becomes more difficult if grief has filled one's life, if deaths of loved ones have left one alone, if lack of mobility constrains one's interactions, or if poverty afflicts one's old age. It is not that it is completely impossible to live well in the face of trouble. Turner suggests, from an Aristotelian perspective, but as the Stoics also argued, that training in virtue throughout life can prepare one to overcome bad luck. Yet it would seem preferable to provide the aging with resources to help them deal with misfortunes they may face so that their lives may go well.

Developing these resources is stymied in part by a third feature of the contemporary picture of the human, its individualism. People in contemporary society are encouraged to work out their problems on their own and develop their own life plans. Life projects are evaluated in terms of their impacts on the individual self and her desires. The continual focus on optimization reinforces this individualism, as one always looks for opportunities to develop and maximize aspects of the self.[6] The medical focus on autonomy, although it started as a defense of patients against unwanted treatments prescribed by doctors, has swiftly become a way of understanding a patient, with bioethicists always fearing the undue influence of family members. As it takes hold, it even shapes understandings of medicine, moving away from ideas of a professional relationship between doctors and patients to that of a service-provider relationship in which medical professionals provide desired treatments in response to individual patients' desires.[7] In this, medicine is starting to embody classical liberal ideals emphasizing individual choice.

Though it is important not to deny the dignity of any person, this emphasis on the individual threatens to obscure essential aspects of what it means to be human, a fact shown by responses to the epidemic of loneliness discussed by Davis. First, this epidemic shows that older adults are experiencing themselves as individuals in the most extreme way, as individuals isolated from others. Second, the responses to this crisis miss the essence of the problem. They focus on the health effects of loneliness or the feelings engendered by loneliness, dreaming of a pill or psychological therapy that will remove these feelings. These palliatives ignore that the problem with loneliness is that humans are not the kind of creatures who are meant to be alone, that communing with others is not merely an instrumental good but is an intrinsic good.

The importance of this insight is shown in Turner's discussion of happiness. Recent research on happiness errs in describing it in terms of subjective emotional states. Instead, happiness as *eudaimonia* must be thought of as an objective state of the person, a condition of the individual that is heavily dependent on the condition of social and political life. As classical philosophy and theology argue, humans are social creatures meant to live in fellowship with others. The possibility that any individual will be happy is shaped by her ability to form meaningful relationships in just social structures. Personhood is not merely posited and developed by the self; it is lived and, in part, constituted through relationships with others.

If one accepts the idea of relational personhood, it follows that improved social relationships can improve the evening of life. Taylor's discussion of friendship and caregiving for people with dementia shows how this can happen. These meaningful social relationships counteract the cognitive and health declines associated with dementia, first by providing concrete care and support. In a broader sense, though, they can counteract such decline by drawing attention away from everyday losses, from the failures to achieve socially mandated optimization, and by refocusing on developing deeper and more valuable relationships with others. The temporal contraction described by Aho aids in this deepening of relationships by older adults. As one sees possibilities for future optimization become more limited, one trims one's obligations and broader networks to focus on and deepen relationships with family and friends. One ceases to be as concerned with elements of life that ultimately do not matter so that one can enrich aspects of true value.

These relationships are not just good for the person suffering decline; they can also help the caregiver develop richer relationships. The chapters by Taylor and by Szanton and Taylor show that, even when engaged with the difficult care of a family member or friend with dementia, caregiving relationships can still enrich the lives of the caregivers. They themselves feel the strength of the connection. The caregiver herself is transformed through the experience, possibly developing new strengths and skills. Of course, this does not diminish the daily difficulties and the frequently overwhelming nature of these caregiving relationships.

It is because of these difficulties faced by caregivers that it is not enough merely to look at individual relationships; there is also a need to develop social mechanisms to support individuals providing care and the relational opportunities of the elderly more broadly. It is of course difficult to transform social institutions focused on individuals to engage the relational self, but some easy first steps are suggested by the authors in this volume. First, there are some straightforward legal and administrative changes that would help people care for friends and neighbors with dementia. Too often, there is a suspicion of nonfamily or even family caregivers, which just creates further obstacles for those already wrestling with difficult situations. Changing the applicable laws and policies in responsible ways will enable people to engage in relational citizenship more easily.

Further changes can take place in regard to the provision of medical care. As Szanton and Taylor argue, medicine needs to shift from a provider/disease-centric model of medicine to a person/community-focused model, mirroring the shift from diagnostic to prognostic medicine supported by Mutter. Such a shift would require programs such as CAPABLE that aim to increase the possibilities for people to engage with their communities by recognizing the functional supports and environmental changes required to allow older adults to get out into communities. Too often, the elderly are prevented from leaving home to engage with others by mobility impairments or the inability to perform tasks of daily life that are the necessary precursors to leaving home. Simple interventions, if they were to become a focus of medicine, would enable individuals to engage in a richer social life. Thus there are simple steps that society can take to aid in the shift from an individualistic to a relational framework.

Ongoing Difficulties

These are good first steps to confront optimization, problematic temporalities, and individualism, but it is important to realize that any such efforts will face strong headwinds and ultimately be ineffective if put forward merely in a piecemeal manner. These efforts are struggling against modernity's underlying vision of the self, which is at the core of the problem of the evening of life. The focus on communities and relationships may falter because they will encounter broad declines in community engagement and social capital. Not only the elderly, but almost all age groups, are encountering others in the offline world less and less.[8] The effort to embrace vulnerability and dependency runs up against the fact that today's young are trained into regimes of self-optimization. Alternative temporalities prove difficult when the pace of life and demands of work are continually speeding up, leaving individuals with little time for savoring the present or the tasks of relational caregiving.⁹ One cannot savor the moment when there is a backlog of emails waiting for responses. To change our engagement with the evening of life requires in some ways that we transform society's understanding of the person, which is obviously a difficult task.

Despite the broad scale of these problems, perhaps aging and dying are exactly the areas in which they can be combated best. These are good points of focus because they are such obvious problems, given the rapid aging of the population and the amount of money spent on programs for the aging. Further, increasing portions of younger populations are struggling with how to care for their aging parents. Therefore, these are sites in which new forms of care, new programs, new understandings can have a broader impact. Efforts to help older adults engage more with the community and to encourage younger people to deepen relationships of care and friendship with those in the evening of life can serve as opportunities to develop broader ties of sociality across the community. Spending time with the vulnerable, especially those with physical and cognitive disabilities, can reframe our understanding of achievement and time. It teaches others how to slow down and learn to enjoy a different pace of life, a pace that is set by another. Finally, caring for the dying forces a person to consider his own end, making each person address this temporal closure. Engaging with the dying puts all attempts at self-optimization in an ultimate perspective. Confronting the problems of people in the evening of life could perhaps enable us to address some of our deepest concerns with our contemporary picture of the human person.

Notes

1. Geoffrey Gorer, "The Pornography of Death," *Encounter* (October 1955): 49–52; Elisabeth Kübler-Ross, *On Death and Dying: What the Dying Have to Teach Doctors, Nurses, Clergy and Their Own Families*, reprint ed. (New York: Scribner, 2014); Ernest Becker, *The Denial of Death* (New York: Free Press, 1973); Philippe Ariès, *The Hour of Our Death*, trans. Helen Weaver (New York: Knopf, 1981); Atul Gawande, *Being Mortal: Medicine and What Matters in the End* (New York: Metropolitan Books, 2014); and The Conversation Project website, 2019, https://theconversationproject.org/.

2. Michel Foucault, *The History of Sexuality*, vol. 1 (New York: Pantheon Books, 1978).

3. For discussion, see President's Council on Bioethics, *Taking Care: Ethical Caregiving in Our Aging Society* (Washington, DC: President's Council on Bioethics, 2005).

4. See also Daniel Callahan, *The Troubled Dream of Life: In Search of a Peaceful Death*, ed. 1 (Washington, DC: Georgetown University Press, 2000).

5. Michel Foucault, *The Hermeneutics of the Subject: Lectures at the Collège de France, 1981-82*, trans. Graham Burchell (New York: Palgrave Macmillan, 2005), 110.

6. However, it is important to note that an emphasis on optimization need not be completely individualistic. Thus, the relentless drive of upper-middle-class parents to maximize their children's educational opportunities and achievements is not strictly individualistic but seeks to optimize the attainments of the family as a social unit. See Michel Foucault, *The Birth of Biopolitics: Lectures at the Collège de France, 1978-79*, ed. Michel Senellart (New York: Palgrave Macmillan, 2008), 227. As neoclassical economists always emphasized, the rational actor can include considerations of others in his calculations of utility. See, for example, Friedrich A. von Hayek, *Individualism and Economic Order* (Chicago: University of Chicago Press, 1948), 13. Still, the regime of optimization, when tied to the current instability of the family and other social institutions, does tend toward individualism.

7. See the critique in Edmund D. Pellegrino, "The Commodification of Medical and Health Care: The Moral Consequences of a Paradigm Shift from a Professional to a Market Ethics," in *The Philosophy of Medicine Reborn: A Pellegrino Reader*, ed. H. Tristram Englehardt and Fabrice Jotterand (Notre Dame, IN: University of Notre Dame Press, 2008).

8. Sherry Turkle, *Alone Together: Why We Expect More from Technology and Less from Each Other* (New York: Basic Books, 2011).

9. Hartmut Rosa, *Social Acceleration: A New Theory of Modernity* (New York: Columbia University Press, 2013).

CONTRIBUTORS

KEVIN AHO is a professor and chair of the Department of Communication and Philosophy at Florida Gulf Coast University. He has published widely in the areas of existentialism, phenomenology, hermeneutics, and the philosophy of medicine. He is the author of *Body Matters: A Phenomenology of Sickness, Illness, and Disease* (with James Aho); *Heidegger's Neglect of the Body*; *Existentialism: An Introduction*; and *Contexts of Suffering: A Heideggerian Approach to Psychopathology*, and editor of *Existential Medicine: Essays on Health and Illness*.

JOSEPH E. DAVIS is a research professor of sociology and moderator of the Picturing the Human colloquy of the Institute for Advanced Studies in Culture at the University of Virginia. His research explores questions of self/identity, morality, and cultural change. In his writing on medicine and psychiatry, he has examined trauma psychology, narratives of suffering, the rise of biological explanations of mental life, medicalization, and psychoactive drug use. His most recent books are *Chemically Imbalanced: Everyday Suffering, Medication, and our Troubled Quest for Self-Mastery*, and, co-edited with Ana Marta González, *To Fix or to Heal: Patient Care, Public Health, and the Limits of Biomedicine*.

CHARLES GUIGNON is emeritus professor of philosophy at the University of South Florida. He is the author of *Heidegger and the Problem of Knowledge*; *On Being Authentic*; and *Re-envisioning Psychology*. He also edited or co-edited *The Cambridge Companion to Heidegger*; *Existentialism: Basic Writings*; *The Existentialists*; *Richard Rorty*; and other books.

SHARON R. KAUFMAN is chair of the Department of Anthropology, History and Social Medicine, University of California, San Francisco. Her work explores topics at the intersection of aging, medical knowledge, and society's expectations for health. She has examined the changing culture and structure of US medicine; health care delivery at the end of life; the relationship of biotechnologies to ethics, governance, and medical practice; and the shifting terrain of evidence in clinical science. She is the author numerous articles and of four books, including *Ordinary Medicine: Extraordinary Treatments, Longer Lives, and Where to Draw the Line*.

WILFRED M. MCCLAY is G. T. and Libby Blankenship Chair in the History of Liberty and director of the Center for the History of Liberty at the University of Oklahoma. He has written widely on the intellectual and cultural history of the United States, with particular attention to the social and political thought of the nineteenth and twentieth centuries and to the history of American religious thought and institutions. Among his books are *The Masterless: Self and Society in Modern America*; *Figures in the Carpet: Finding the Human Person in the American Past*; *Why Place Matters: Geography, Identity, and Civic Life in Modern America*; and *Land of Hope: An Invitation to the Great American Story*.

JUSTIN MUTTER is an assistant professor of family medicine and geriatric medicine at the University of Virginia School of Medicine. He also serves as core faculty in the School of Medicine's Center for Biomedical Ethics and Humanities and is a fellow at the Institute for Advanced Studies in Culture. He obtained his MD at the University of Virginia and completed graduate work in the history of science, medicine, and technology at the University of Oxford. His clinical, teaching, and research interests lie at the intersection of person-centered care, health policy for older adults, and the modern history of American medicine and public health.

PAUL SCHERZ is an associate professor of moral theology and ethics at the Catholic University of America; co-chair of the Joint Masters Program in Catholic Clinical Ethics with Georgetown University's Pellegrino Center for Clinical Bioethics; and a visiting faculty fellow at the Institute for Advanced Studies in Culture. His research, drawing on his dual trainings in theology (Notre Dame) and molecular biology (Harvard), examines the interrelationship between ethics, religion, science, technology, and medicine. He has published widely in both science and theology; his publications include his book *Science and Christian Ethics*.

SARAH L. SZANTON is a professor and director of the Center for Innovative Care in Aging at the Johns Hopkins School of Nursing. She holds a joint appointment in the Department of Health Policy and Management at the Johns Hopkins Bloomberg School of Public Health. She tests interventions to reduce health disparities among older adults. Her work particularly focuses on ways to help older adults "age in place," including modifying housing, improving access to food, and other initiatives to improve the social determinants of health. Among other sources, her work has been funded by the National Institutes of Health, the Center for Medicare and Medicaid Services Innovation Center, and the Robert Wood Johnson Foundation.

JANELLE S. TAYLOR is a medical anthropologist and professor of anthropology at the University of Toronto. Her current research focuses on dementia, with special attention given to the importance of social relationships beyond the family and the situations of older adults with dementia who do not have family available to provide caregiving support.

JANIECE TAYLOR is an assistant professor in the School of Nursing and principal faculty in the Center for Innovative Care in Aging at Johns Hopkins University. She received her doctorate from the University of Texas at Austin, where she received training in disability research and minority aging research. Her dissertation focused on predictors of disability among middle-aged and older African American women with osteoarthritis.

BRYAN S. TURNER is emeritus professor of sociology at the Graduate Center, City University of New York; honorary professor of sociology at Potsdam University; and professor of sociology at the Australian Catholic University, Melbourne, Australia. In 2015, he won the Max Planck Award. He holds a doctor of letters degree from the University of Cambridge. With a background in the sociology of the body, he has been interested in problems of human vulnerability. His recent publications in this field include *Can We Live Forever?*; *L'antivieillissement: Vieillir à l'ère des nouvelles biotechnologies* (with Alex Dumas); and a special issue of *The Sociological Quarterly* on "Human Longevity, Utopia and Solidarity" (with Alex Dumas).

INDEX

acceleration (*Schnelligkeit*), 86
activities of daily living (ADLs), 148, 152, 153–54, 156
Adams, Rachel, 140
"adaptive perspective" of health and illness, 175
addiction, impact on life expectancy, 116
adolescence, extension of, 181
Adult Protective Services, 139
advanced directives, 50, 185
aged. *See* elderly
ageism, 79–81, 92n2, 94–95, 165
aging
    and advances in medical science, 107–8
    avoidance of, 29, 46, 48
    as beginning, 87
    and embodiment, 108, 115–16
    as an engineering problem, 108
    epiphanies of, 68
    fear of, 68
    humor of, 67
    as liberation from ideas of permanence and self-subsistence, 89
    as loss of self-sufficiency and autonomy, 111–12
    medicalization of, 6, 18n26, 24
    negative age stereotypes, 18n26
    and norms of middle age, 182
    not a problem to be solved, 77
    opportunities for personal and spiritual growth, 9
    optimistic views of, 114–17
    as "other," 6
    in popular culture, 24, 25–28
    psychological problems of, 108
    and role of family, 52
    science of, 28–30, 164, 175
    as temporal contraction, 81–84
    See also old age
"aging in place," 147–48
aging of the population, 4–5, 18n26, 191
Aho, Kevin, 6, 9, 10, 184, 185
Allen, Woody, 68
Allison, Anne, 129
Alzheimer's disease, 12, 57
    as diagnostic entity, 163
    fast growing numbers living with, 5

Alzheimer's disease (*cont.*)
　as loss of selfhood, 12, 125
　as a vocation, 57
American Association of Retired Persons (AARP), 23
American healthcare, capitalistic practices of, 163, 165
Améry, Jean, 95, 96–98
anthropology of ethics, 48
anti-aging therapies, 2, 28–30
appetite (*epithumia*), 113
Aristotle, 10–11, 105–6, 107, 115–16
　on aging and death, 47, 112–14
　on *eudaimonia*, 108–12
　on wisdom of elderly, 118–19
ars moriendi tradition, 59
assisted suicide, 2, 51
Auschwitz, 96
authenticity
　and aging, 78–79, 80, 84, 90–91, 101–3, 184–85
　and moral values, 104n18
　as resoluteness, 89
autonomy, 5, 7, 26–27, 47–49, 111, 119
　and bioethics, 52
　cannot answer the issues of old age, 50
　and citizenship, 138–39, 140–41
　and hospice care, 52
　medical focus on, 188
　See also individualism

Baby Boomer generation, graying of, 165
Bagley, Nicholas, 174
Baltes, Margret, 117
Banner, Michael, 51–52, 57, 63n36
Becker, Ernest, 80

behavioral activation, 151–52, 156, 157
Bellarmine, Robert, 59
belongingness, 99
Bennett, Tony, 94
Benny, Jack, 67
bioethics, focus on autonomy, 52
biomedical research, 41, 168
biomedicine, 8, 162–63
　atomization of, 170
biotechnology, 168
bodily strength, decay of, 31
Botox, 29
Brin, Sergey, 95
Brown, E. Richard, 163
Brown, Lawrence, 175
Buber, Martin, 87
Buddhism, 57–58, 59
burdening others, 51, 52

Cacioppo, John, 32, 36n27
Cacioppo, Stephanie, 32, 36n27
care and solidarity, undermined social basis for, 30
caregivers, 11, 12–13, 127–29, 189–90, 191
　informal, 127–29
　nonkin, 128–29
　See also family caregivers; person-centered care
Carstensen, Laura, 107, 117–18
Cassel, Christine, 174
Catholic Church, on preparation for death, 59
Catholic spirituality, 56
Centers for Medicare and Medicaid Services, 166
character, 48
children, vulnerability of, 53

Christ, emptying of self, 55
Christianity, on humility, dependence, and vulnerability, 55
chronic pain, 115
Cicero, 54, 58, 103
citizenship
　premised on autonomy, 138–39, 140–41
　and relational personhood, 137–42
　as sociality, 141
clinical knowledge, 131
clinical medicine, 41–42
community
　and aging, 13, 147–49, 190
　collective approach to dementia, 131–32
Community Aging in Place, Advancing Better Living for Elders (CAPABLE) Program, 148, 152–57, 184, 190
connectedness, of well-lived life, 101
Conrad, Peter, 169
consequentialist ethics, 46–47
Consolidated Omnibus Reconciliation Act (COBRA), 162, 176
Croce, Benedetto, 107
"cultural time," 97–98
Cumming, Elaine, 113
curiosity (*Neugier*), 82
Curtis, Jamie Lee, 26–27

Dasein, 81–82, 89, 99–100
Davis, Bette, 106, 118
Davis, Joseph, 6, 181, 182, 185, 188
death, 185
　avoidance of, 51, 52, 59
　as choice, 186
　considered premature, 41, 186
　hiddenness of dying, 185
　meditation on, 53, 57–59
　preparing for, 59
　as temporal closure, 184–86
　See also assisted suicide; dying well
death anxiety, 80–81
death awareness program, 185
de Beauvoir, Simone, 90, 97
Deci, Edward, 107
"default surrogate consent statutes," 139
de Grey, Aubrey, 108, 118
dementia
　and caregiving, 12–13
　as death before death, 57
　framing talk about, 131–32
　and friendship, 129–32
　healthcare costs, 173
　as loss of personhood, 63n36, 125–26, 128
　and personal transformation, 130–31
　and personhood, 129, 131
　talking about, 25, 131–32, 136
　See also Alzheimer's disease
deontological ethics, 47
dependency, 34, 48, 52, 53–57, 190
depression, 154, 155–56
Desjarlais, Robert, 57–58
diagnosis
　as narrowly biomedical, 162–63
　political economy of, 163–65, 166, 168–69, 170, 173, 184
　tyranny, 183
diagnosis-related groups (DRGs), 166–67, 168, 169, 173
diagnostic coding, 168
diagnostic regime, 169, 173, 183
dignity, 5, 51, 54, 157, 188
disability becomes strength, 68, 72
disengagement theory, 112–13

divorce rate, among aged, 32
Donnellan, M. Brent, 119
drugs, and aging, 108
dying well, 2, 57–59

elderly
  dehumanizing of, 81
  epithets for, 95
  loneliness of, 31–33
  as strangers to the world, 97
  as whole persons, 170
  wisdom of, 95, 118–19
Elias, Norbert, 31, 36n21
embodiment, 11, 53, 55
  and aging, 13–14, 118–19
emotivism, 106
endless existence, 108, 118
end-of-life care, 49, 51
"engineered negligible senescence," 2
epidemic of loneliness. *See* loneliness: epidemic of
Erasmus, 59
ethic of life extension, 43–44
ethics of aging, 2–3, 4
Etzioni, Amitai, 106
eudaimonia, 105, 107, 108–12, 188
evening of the body as morning of the spirit, 76
everydayness, 98, 99
evidence-based medicine, 41, 45
existentialism, 96
existential time, 82
extraordinary care, 50

families
  and communities and aging, 117
  of persons with dementia, 137
  strengthened by daily care of family members, 151

family caregivers, 5, 127–29
fear of aging, 5–6
feminist ethics of care, 11, 54
Finkelstein, Amy, 169
flourishing. *See* human flourishing
forbearance, 10
Foucault, Michel, 185, 187
frailty, 14
frailty syndrome, 171–73
Freud, Sigmund, 107
friendship, 16, 129–30
  and abandonment, 132–37
  with persons with dementia, 137, 189–90
functional imperative, 170–73
future, 96
  as a contracting horizon, 17, 79, 82, 88, 117, 185
  as open and indefinite, 100–101, 185

Gawande, Atul, 18n29
Gelassenheit (letting be), 102
generativity, in late life, 149
geriatric medicine, 14, 170–71
giftedness of life, 54
goal setting, 151, 153–56, 157
Golden Rule, 54
Gorer, Geoffrey, 185
Graeber, David, 137
Gratton, Brian, 168
"gray divorce," 32
Greenberg, Jeff, 81
guardian ad litem, 139
Guignon, Charles, 10, 184

Haber, Carole, 168
Hadot, Pierre, 58
Hall, Donald, 9

happiness, 105, 188–89
  as consumption, 111, 114
  as contentment, 106, 109, 115, 118
  as an illusion, 107
  and pleasure, 114
  as political and social, 114, 118
  as private experience, 106–7
  and virtue, 110–12, 115
  and wealth, 114, 116
Harriot, Howard H., 112
health, "non-health" factors in, 149
health and fitness, and devaluation of old age, 27
healthcare, 4–5
  for older adults, 164
  private industry in, 40, 41
health insurance for the elderly, 24
hedonism, 107
Heidegger, Martin, 58, 81–84, 86, 88–90, 95, 98–102, 185
Henry, William Earl, 113
hospice care, 39, 51, 52
human flourishing, 11, 16, 103
  in aging, 106
  and community of others, 53
  and political life, 105–6, 107, 111, 114
humans
  age of wholeness, 72
  as dependent rational animals, 53–54
  ergon of, 109
  as social creatures, 8, 99, 189
humility, 55–56, 59, 184
Husserl, Edmund, 98

identity, 125
Illich, Ivan, 30
immortality, 5

implantable cardioverter defibrillators (ICDs), 42–45
inauthenticity
  of ageist stereotypes, 91
  as denial of vulnerability, 88–89
individualism, 5, 28, 34, 188–89. *See also* autonomy
instrumental activities of daily living (IADLs), 152
interdependence, 28, 140
invasive care options, 50
Islam, dependence on God, 55

Jacobs, Lawrence, 167
John Paul II (pope), Parkinson's disease, 56
joy, of aging, 76
Judaism, dependence on God, 55
Jung, Carl, 33

Kahn, Robert, 28, 32
Kant, Immanuel, 47
Kar-Purkayastha, Ishani, 37n30
Katz, Stephen, 24
Kaufman, Sharon, 6–7, 15, 47, 49, 186
kenosis, 55–56
Khosla, Vinod, 79
Kierkegaard, Søren, 3

Laslett, Peter, 107
left ventricular assist device (LVAD), 45
Levitsky, Sandra, 127
life expectancy
  and addiction, 116
  and advances in medical science, 115
  and reflection on contracting future, 83
life-extending treatments, 39–45, 108

lifeworld, 99
Lindemann, Hilde, 138
lived time, 96
living old age well, 8–11
living slowly, 86–88
living wills, 50
Lock, Margaret, 116
loneliness
   epidemic of, 25, 31–33, 188
   as problem to be solved, 37n31
loss becomes gain, 72
love, 39
Lucas, Richard E., 119

MacIntyre, Alasdair, 53, 106, 107
Manning, Margaret, 25–27
martyrdom, 57
Mattingly, Cheryl, 130
Mayes, Rick, 166
May, Theresa, 37n31
McClay, Wilfred, 9, 10, 184
McKnight, Robin, 169
medical-industrial complex, 163, 167
medicalization of lives of older adults, 6, 24
medical jurisdiction, over "nonmedical" problems, 169
Medicare, 163–64, 165–66, 173
   as fiscal program, 174–75
   funding of, 42, 52, 184
   incrementalism of, 167–68
   use of diagnosis, 14, 166–69
Medicare Wellness Visit, 148
medicine
   ability to prolong wanted life, 39
   disease-centric model, 190
   does not attend to suffering, 39
   as instrumental problem-solving, 6
   person/community-focused model, 190

meditation on death, 53, 57–59
Mencken, H. L., 73, 76
middle age, governing norms of, 181–82
Midgley, Mary, 30
midlife crisis, 83, 91
Montaigne, 58
moods (*Stimmungen*), 100
Moody, Harry, 25
Murthy, Vivek, 32
Mutter, Justin, 14, 183, 190

narrative cohesion, 16, 90
Nascher, Ignatz Leo, 170
nearness (*die Nähe*), 86
Neuberger, Richard, 85
"new gerontology," 28–30
"new immortalist movement," 30
new technologies, and timing of death, 41
Nietzsche, Friedrich, 107
"noncontractarian account of care," 140
Nussbaum, Martha, 108–9, 140–41

O'Connor, John (cardinal), 52
old age
   amorphousness of, 181
   commercialization of, 24
   as cultural category, 3
   debilities of, 71
   embodiment in, 118–19
   inner development during, 74
   no value in itself, 30
   positive conceptions of, 2–3
   roles and identities appropriate for, 34
   romanticized in pre-modern cultures, 95
   as sharpening of awareness, 87

as social problem, 3–7
and strengthening of social
  relations, 34
as virtuous living, 187
older adults. *See* elderly
Older Americans Act (1965), 165
Olson, Laura, 165
open future, as inauthentic existence,
  185–87
opioid addiction, 116
optimized self. *See* self-optimization
organ transplants, 186
overtreatment, at end of life, 51

Page, Larry, 95
pain and motivation, 155–56
pain management, 118
"paradox of well-being," 9, 91
patience, 54
Patient Self-Determination Act
  (1990), 50
person-centered care, 14, 151, 170,
  175, 176
personhood
  as autonomy, 2, 60
  as individually oriented, 12, 126,
    188
  as relational, 12, 16, 126, 130, 142,
    189–90
  social practices of, 138
  and supportive environment, 13
  See also selfhood
persons with dementia
  abandonment of, 138
  friendship with, 132–37
  interaction with, 131
  living alone, 128
  vulnerable to exploitation, 134–35
phenomenology, 98. *See also*
  Heidegger, Martin

Pinker, Steven, 107, 111, 114–17,
  118, 119
Plato, 58
Pols, Jeannette, 141–42
Portacolone, Elena, 129
potentiality, 3, 88
power of attorney, 139
power in weakness, 9, 68, 76
principlism, 7, 48
proceduralism, 7, 47
professional guardians, 139–40
prognosis, political economy of,
  175–76, 184
prospective payment system (PPS),
  166–67

"quality of life," 76
Quinlan, Karen Ann, 49

Rae, Michael, 108
Reagan, Ronald, 166
rebound. *See* resilience
Reinhardt, Uwe, 169
Reiser, Stanley, 175
relational citizenship, 137–42
resignation, 96, 102
resilience, 149–51, 155
resistance, 10
resoluteness (*Entschlossenheit*), 89,
  90, 101–2
restlessness, 86, 91
restorative medicine, 29
reverence, in later life, 102–3
revolt, of old age, 101–2
risks, treatment of, 42
Rosenberg, Charles E., 38, 162–63,
  164, 168
Rowe, John, 28, 32
Royce, Josiah, 112
Ryan, Richard, 107

Samuel, Lawrence, 164–65
Saunders, Cicely, 52
Scherz, Paul, 7, 8, 10
self-coherence, and aging process, 90
selfhood
  and active caregivers, 12
  as individual, 182
  meaning from the look of another, 96
  modernity's vision of, 190
  as relational, 182
  and supportive networks, 126
self-optimization, 28, 182–83, 186–87, 188, 190, 192n6
self-sufficiency, 109, 111
  and assisted suicide, 51
Simmel, George, 18n25, 19n35
slowness, as liberating, 86–88, 91
Smith, Christian, 111
social capital, 190
socialization, 100
social obligation, 39
Social Security, 5, 165–66, 168
social time, 97
Society to Cells Resilience Framework, 149–51
Socioemotional Selectivity Theory (SST), 84–85
sociology, as modern dismal science, 115
spiritedness (*thumos*), 113
steadfastness, 101
stinginess, 112
Stoicism, 48, 58, 187
"strange relationships," with persons with dementia, 134–35, 137
"successful aging," 2, 6, 8, 25, 27, 28–30, 147, 182–83

suffering
  and finitude, 89
  value in, 8, 60
Szanton, Sarah, 13–14, 189, 190

Taylor, Charles, 130
Taylor, Janelle, 12–13, 57, 182
Taylor, Janiece, 14, 189, 190
technocratic corporatism, 175
temporal contraction, 79, 81–84
temporality, 9, 16, 100–101, 190
Terror Management Theory (TMT), 80–81
time, 70, 81–82
Tinetti, Mary, 170
tragedy, endurance through, 131
Turner, Bryan, 10–11, 187, 188

United Nations Convention on the Rights of Persons with Disabilities (UNCRPD), 140
utilitarianism, 7, 46, 107, 109

Varga, Somogy, 104n18
Viagra, 29
Vincent, John, 3
virtue, 10–11, 48
  and happiness, 105
  training in, 188
volunteer guardians, 140
vulnerability, 3, 14, 109, 140, 190
  blindness to reality of, 183–85
  of the body, 109
  at core of human condition, 53–56, 85–86, 88–89
  of elderly, 88–89, 34
  to stressors, 171–72

Ware, Bronnie, 78
weakness, 9, 60, 68, 76
Weber, Max, 106, 107
well-lived life, 34
whole-person care. *See* person-centered care
widow and orphan, 54
will of God, 59

wisdom, in late life, 149
wonder, 9, 54, 87, 186

Yalom, Irvin, 89
Yeats, William Butler, 9, 71, 75–76
youth culture, 94

Zuckerberg, Mark, 79, 95

www.ingramcontent.com/pod-product-compliance
Lightning Source LLC
Chambersburg PA
CBHW030623230426
43661CB00053B/2121